GW01377296

Plant Based Diet Cookbook 2021

2 Books in 1: A Collection of 100+ Healthy Plant-Based Recipes for Losing Weight and Feeling Great

Frank Smith

© Copyright 2021 - All rights reserved.

The content contained within this book may not be reproduced, duplicated or transmitted without direct written permission from the author or the publisher.

Under no circumstances will any blame or legal responsibility be held against the publisher, or author, for any damages, reparation, or monetary loss due to the information contained within this book. Either directly or indirectly.

Legal Notice:

This book is copyright protected. This book is only for personal use. You cannot amend, distribute, sell, use, quote or paraphrase any part, or the content within this book, without the consent of the author or publisher.

Disclaimer Notice:

Please note the information contained within this document is for educational and entertainment purposes only. All effort has been executed to present accurate, up to date, and reliable, complete information. No warranties of any kind are declared or implied. Readers acknowledge that the author is not engaging in the rendering of legal, financial, medical or professional advice. The content within this book has been derived from various sources. Please consult a licensed professional before attempting any techniques outlined in this book.

By reading this document, the reader agrees that under no circumstances is the author responsible for any losses, direct or indirect, which are incurred as a result of the use of information contained within this document, including, but not limited to, errors, omissions, or inaccuracies.

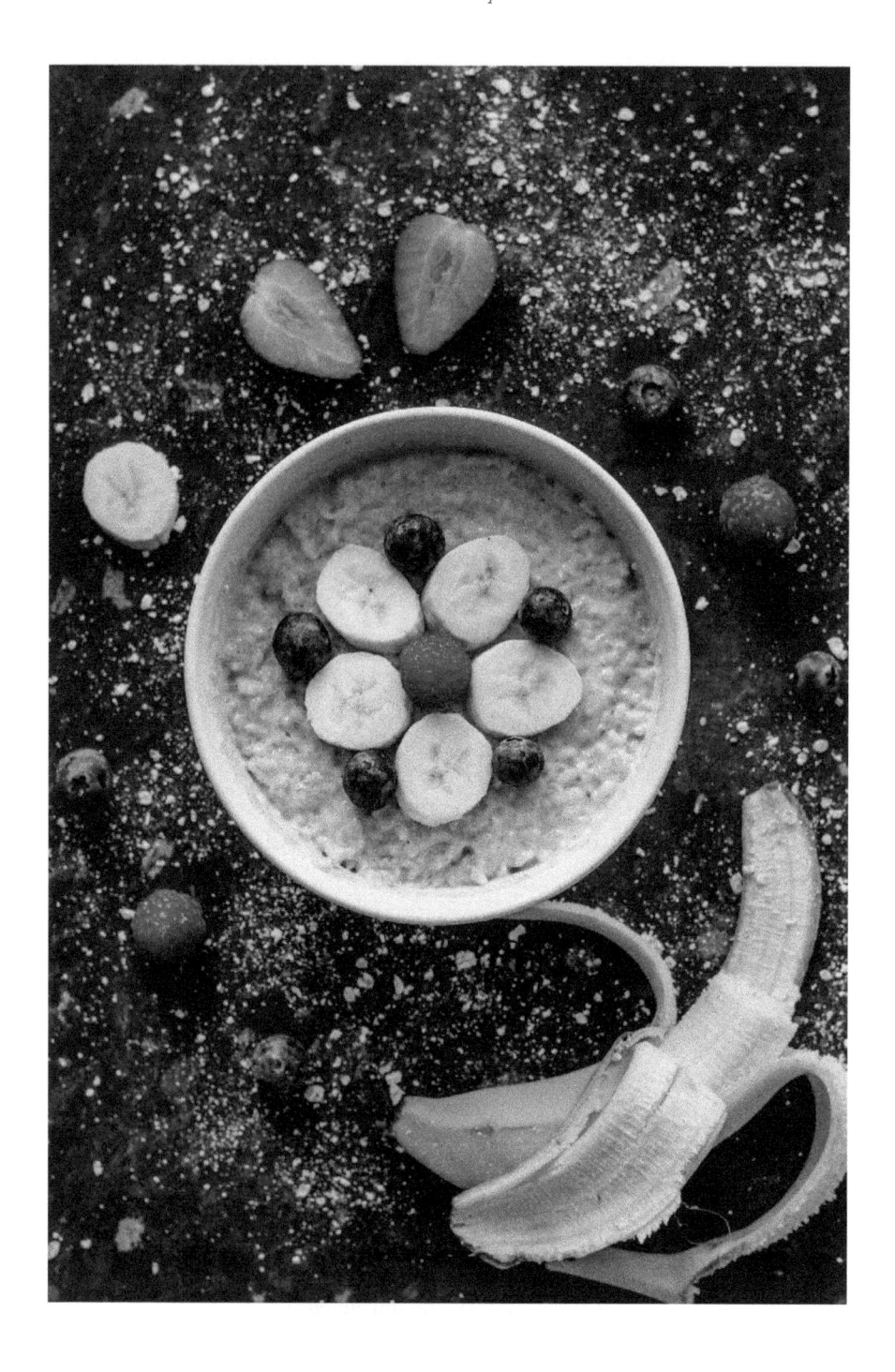

Plant Based Diet Recipes 2021

Plant Based Diet Recipes 2021

A Collection of Healthy Plant-Based Recipes for Losing Weight and Healthy Eating

Frank Smith

Table Of Contents

BREAKFASTS **10**

1. ONION & MUSHROOM TART WITH A NICE BROWN RICE CRUST 10
2. PERFECT BREAKFAST SHAKE 13
3. BEET GAZPACHO 14
4. HEALTHY BREAKFAST BOWL 16
5. PUMPKIN PANCAKES 17
6. GREEN BREAKFAST SMOOTHIE 18
7. BLUEBERRY AND CHIA SMOOTHIE 19
8. BERRIES WITH MASCARPONE ON TOASTED BREAD 20
9. FRUIT CUP 21
10. OATMEAL WITH BLACK BEANS & CHEDDAR 22
11. STRAWBERRY SMOOTHIE BOWL 23

SOUPS, SALADS, AND SIDES **25**

12. CREAMY SQUASH SOUP 25
13. CUCUMBER EDAMAME SALAD 27
14. BEST BROCCOLI SALAD 29

ENTRÉES **30**

15. CRUNCHY ASPARAGUS SPEARS 30
16. CUCUMBER BITES WITH CHIVE AND SUNFLOWER SEEDS 32

SMOOTHIES AND BEVERAGES **34**

17. TANGY SPICED CRANBERRY DRINK 34
18. WARM POMEGRANATE PUNCH 36
19. RICH TRUFFLE HOT CHOCOLATE 37
20. VANILLA MILKSHAKE 38
21. RASPBERRY PROTEIN SHAKE 39
22. RASPBERRY ALMOND SMOOTHIE 40
23. APPLE RASPBERRY COBBLER 41

SNACKS AND DESSERTS **42**

24. SIMPLE BANANA FRITTERS 42
25. COCONUT AND BLUEBERRIES ICE CREAM 44
26. PEACH CROCKPOT PUDDING 45
27. GREEN SOY BEANS HUMMUS 46
28. HIGH PROTEIN AVOCADO GUACAMOLE 48
29. HOMEMADE ENERGY NUT BARS 49
30. CHOCOLATE ENERGY SNACK BAR 50
31. ZESTY ORANGE MUFFINS 51

| 32 | Chocolate Tahini Balls | 52 |

DINNER RECIPES 54

| 33 | Piquillo Salsa Verde Steak | 54 |
| 34 | Sweet 'n spicy tofu | 56 |

LUNCH RECIPES 57

35	Green Pea Fritters	57
36	Broccoli Rabe	59
37	Whipped Potatoes	60
38	Chickpea Avocado Sandwich	61
39	Pizza Bites	62
40	Avocado, Spinach and Kale Soup	63
41	Curry spinach soup	64
42	Hot roasted peppers cream	65

RECIPES FOR MAIN COURSES AND SINGLE DISHES 67

43	Smoked Tempeh with Broccoli Fritters	67
44	Cheesy Potato Casserole	70
45	Curry Mushroom Pie	71

NUTRIENT-PACKED PROTEIN SALADS 74

| 46 | Arugula Lentil Salad | 74 |

FLAVOUR BOOSTERS (FISH GLAZES, MEAT RUBS & FISH RUBS) ... 77

| 47 | Tunisian Mixed Spiced Rub | 77 |
| 48 | All Purpose Dill Seed Rub | 79 |

SAUCE RECIPES 81

| 49 | Vegan Ranch Dressing (Dipping Sauce) | 81 |
| 50 | Vegan Smokey Maple BBQ Sauce | 83 |

BREAKFASTS 86

51	Oatmeal Fruit Shake	86
52	Amaranth Banana Breakfast Porridge	88
53	Green Ginger Smoothie	89
54	Chocolate Strawberry Almond Protein Smoothie	90
55	Apple and Cinnamon Oatmeal	91
56	13 bis. Mango Key Lime Pie Smoothie	92
57	Spiced Orange Breakfast Couscous	93
58	Fig & Cheese Oatmeal	94
59	Pumpkin Oats	95
60	Apple Chia Pudding	96

SOUPS, SALADS, AND SIDES 97
- 61 GARDEN PATCH SANDWICHES ON MULTIGRAIN BREAD 97
- 62 GARDEN SALAD WRAPS 99
- 63 MARINATED MUSHROOM WRAPS 101

ENTRÉES 104
- 64 HOMEMADE TRAIL MIX 104
- 65 NUT BUTTER MAPLE DIP 105

SMOOTHIES AND BEVERAGES 106
- 66 KALE & AVOCADO SMOOTHIE 106
- 67 COCONUT & STRAWBERRY SMOOTHIE 108
- 68 PUMPKIN CHIA SMOOTHIE 109
- 69 MINI BERRY TARTS 110
- 70 MIXED NUT CHOCOLATE FUDGE 112
- 71 DATE CAKE SLICES 113
- 72 CHOCOLATE MOUSSE CAKE 115

SNACKS AND DESSERTS 117
- 73 NORI SNACK ROLLS 117
- 74 RISOTTO BITES 119
- 75 JICAMA AND GUACAMOLE 120
- 76 OVEN-BAKED CARAMELIZE PLANTAINS 121
- 77 POWERFUL PEAS & LENTILS DIP 122
- 78 PROTEIN "RAFFAELLO" CANDIES 123
- 79 ROASTED CAULIFLOWER 124

DINNER RECIPES 126
- 80 CAULIFLOWER STEAK KICKING CORN 126
- 81 GREEN BEANS STIR FRY 128
- 82 MEAN BEAN MINESTRONE 129

LUNCH RECIPES 132
- 83 CHICKPEA AND EDAMAME SALAD 132
- 84 CAULIFLOWER SALAD 134
- 85 GARLIC MASHED POTATOES & TURNIPS 136
- 86 PULLED "PORK" SANDWICHES 137
- 87 COCONUT ZUCCHINI CREAM 139
- 88 ZUCCHINI AND CAULIFLOWER SOUP 140
- 89 CHARD SOUP 141
- 90 EGGPLANT AND OLIVES STEW 142

RECIPES FOR MAIN COURSES AND SINGLE DISHES 143

91	PECAN & BLUEBERRY CRUMBLE	143
92	RICE PUDDING	145

NUTRIENT-PACKED PROTEIN SALADS 147

93	CHICKPEA, RED KIDNEY BEAN AND FETA SALAD	147
94	CURRIED CARROT SLAW WITH TEMPEH	149
95	BLACK & WHITE BEAN QUINOA SALAD	151
96	GREEK SALAD WITH SEITAN GYROS STRIPS	153
97	CHICKPEA AND EDAMAME SALAD	154

FLAVOUR BOOSTERS (FISH GLAZES, MEAT RUBS & FISH RUBS) . 156

98	MEXICAN COCOA RUB	156
99	JUNIPER SAGE MEAT RUB	158

SAUCE RECIPES 160

100	COCONUT SUGAR PEANUT SAUCE	160

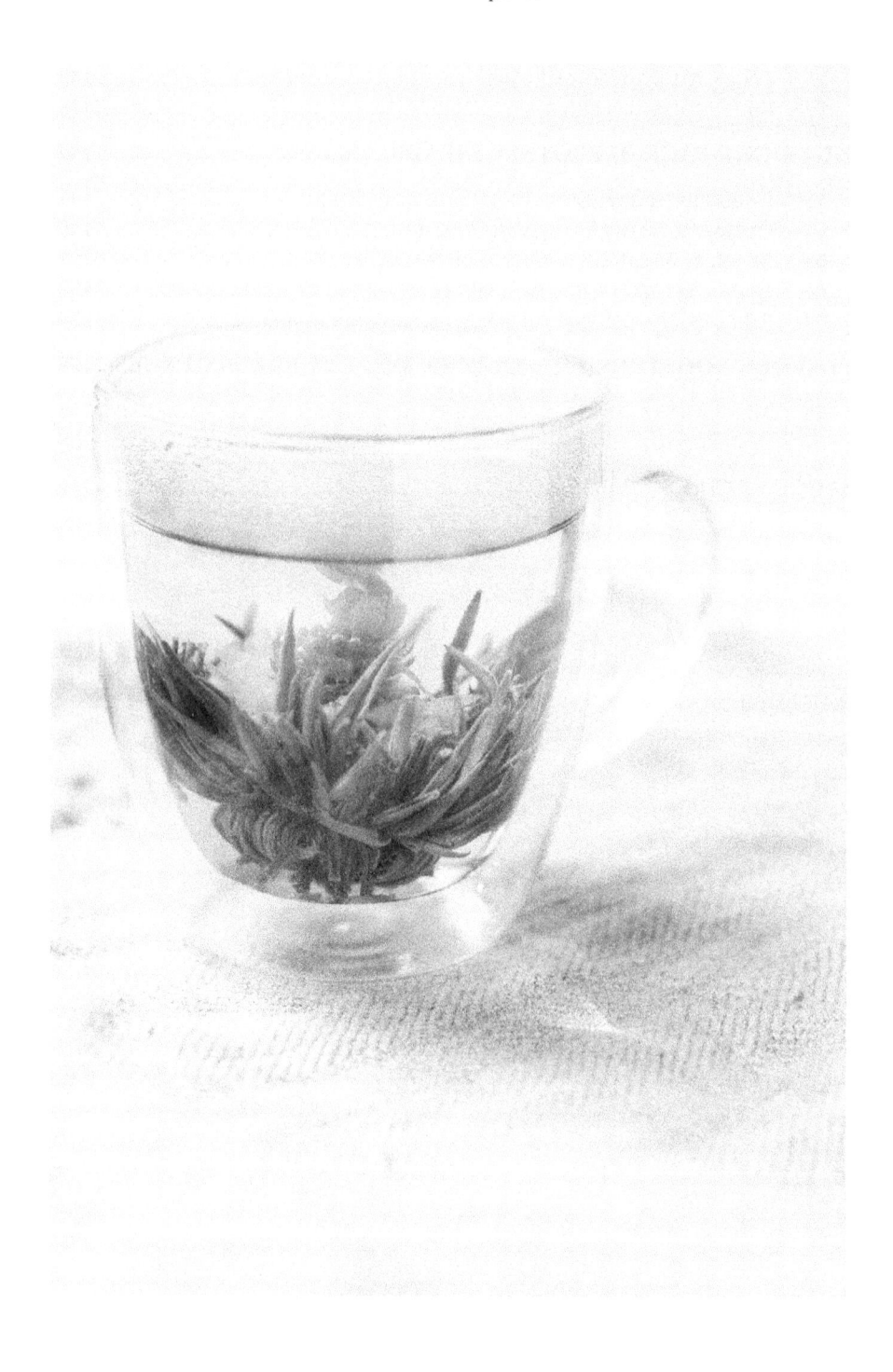

Breakfasts

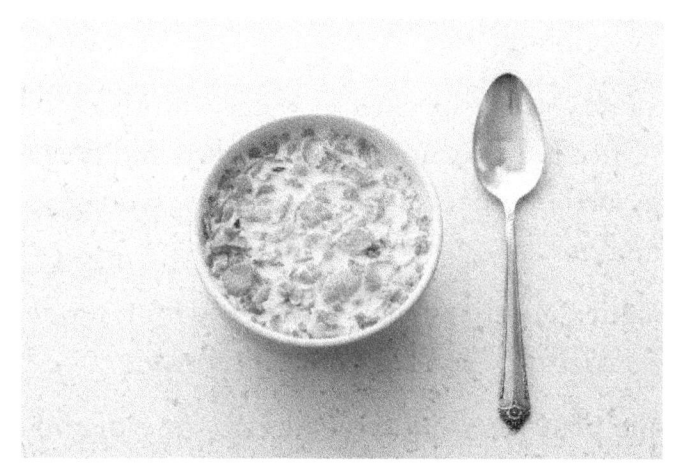

1 Onion & Mushroom Tart with a Nice Brown Rice Crust

Preparation 10 minutesCooking 55 minutes Serving: 1
Ingredients:

1 ½ pounds, mushrooms, button, portabella,1 cup, short-grain brown rice

2 ¼ cups, water

½ teaspoon, ground black pepper 2 teaspoons, herbal spice blend 1 sweet large onion 7 ounces, extra-firm tofu

1 cup, plain non-dairy milk 2 teaspoons, onion powder

2 teaspoons, low-sodium soy1 teaspoon, molasses
¼ teaspoon, ground turmeric ¼ cup, white wine

¼ cup, tapiocaDirections:
Cook the brown rice and put it aside for later use.

Slice the onions into thin strips and sauté them in water until they are soft. Then, add the molasses, and cook them for a few minutes.

Next, sauté the mushrooms in water with the herbal spice blend. Once the mushrooms are cooked and they are soft, add the white wine or sherry. Cook everything for a few more minutes.

In a blender, combine milk, tofu, arrowroot, turmeric, and onion powder till you have a smooth mixture

On a pie plate, create a layer of rice, spreading evenly to form a crust. The rice should be warm and not cold. It will be easy to work with warm rice. You can also use a pastry roller to get an even crust. With your fingers, gently press the sides.

Take half of the tofu mixture and the mushrooms and spoon them over the tart dish. Smooth the level with your spoon.

Now, top the layer with onions followed by the tofu mixture. You can smooth the surface again with your spoon.

Sprinkle some black pepper on top.

Bake the pie at 350o F for about 45 minutes. Toward the end, you can cover it loosely with tin foil. This will help the crust to remain moist.

Allow the pie crust to cool down, so that you can slice it. If you are in love with vegetarian dishes, there is no way that you will not love thispie.

Nutrition: Calories: 245.3, Fats 16.4 g, Proteins 6.8 g, Carbohydrates 18.3 g

2 Perfect Breakfast Shake

Preparation: 5 minutesCooking: 0 minutes Servings: 2
Ingredients:

3 tablespoons, raw cacao powder1 cup, almond milk
2 frozen bananas

3 tablespoons, natural peanut butterDirections:
Use a powerful blender to combine all the ingredients. Process everything until you have a smooth shake.
Enjoy a hearty shake to kickstart your day.

Nutrition: Calories: 330, Fats 15 g, Carbohydrates 41 g, Proteins 11g

3 Beet Gazpacho

Preparation time: 10 minutes Cooking time: 2 minutes
Servings: 4
Ingredients:

½ large bunch young beets with stems, roots and leaves 2 small cloves garlic, peeled,
Salt to taste

Pepper to taste

½ teaspoon liquid stevia 1 glass coconut milk kefir 1 teaspoon chopped dill
½ tablespoon canola oil

1 small red onion, chopped

1 tablespoon apple cider vinegar 2 cups vegetable broth or water 1 tablespoon chopped chives
1 scallion, sliced Roasted baby potatoes Directions:
Cut the roots and stems of the beets into small pieces. Thinly slice the beet greens.

Place a saucepan over medium heat. Add oil. When the oil is heated, add onion and garlic and cook until onion turns translucent.

Stir in the beets, roots and stem and cook for a minute.

Add broth, salt and water and cover with a lid. Simmer until tender.

Add stevia and vinegar and mix well. Taste and adjust the

stevia andvinegar if required.

Turn off the heat. Blend with an immersion blender until smooth.

Place the saucepan back over it. When it begins to boil, add beetgreens and cook for a minute. Turn off the heat.

Cool completely. Chill if desired. Add rest of the ingredients and stir.
Serve in bowls with roasted potatoes if desired.

Nutrition: Calories 101, Fats 5 g, Carbohydrates 14 g, Proteins 2 g

4 Healthy Breakfast Bowl

Preparation: 10 mCooking: 10 m Ingredients:

1 vegan yogurt 1/2 avocado (peeled and diced) 1 handful blueberries 1 tablespoon cacao nibs 1 handful of strawberries 1 tablespoon mulberries 1 tablespoon goji berries tablespoon desiccated coconut

1 Directions:

Put the avocado in a nice bowl. Top up with vegan yogurt.

Sprinkle the remaining ingredients and enjoy it.

Nutrition: carbohydrates: 55 g calories: 471 Fat: 25g sodium: 183 gprotein: 11 g sugar: 32 g

5 Pumpkin Pancakes

Preparation time: 15 minutes Cooking time: 15 minutes
Servings: 4
Ingredients

1 cups unsweetened almond milk 1 teaspoon apple cider vinegar 2½ cups whole-wheat flour
2 tablespoons baking powder

½ Teaspoon baking soda 1 teaspoon sea salt
1 teaspoon pumpkin pie spice or ½ teaspoon ground cinnamon plus ¼ teaspoon grated nutmeg plus ¼ teaspoon ground allspice ½ Cup canned pumpkin purée 1 cup water tablespoon coconut oil Directions
In a small bowl, combine the almond milk and apple cider vinegar. Set aside.

In a bowl, whisk together the flour, baking powder, baking soda, salt, and pumpkin pie spice. In bowl, combine the almond milk mixture, pumpkin purée, and water, whisking to mix well. Mix the wet Ingredients to the dry Ingredients and fold together until the dry- Ingredients are just moistened.

In a nonstick pan or griddle over medium-high heat, melt the coconut oil and swirl to coat. Pour the batter into the pan ¼ cup at a time and cook until the pancakes are browned, about 5 minutes per side. Serve immediately.

6 Green Breakfast Smoothie

Preparation: 10 minutesCooking: 0 minutes Servings: 2
Ingredients

½ Banana, sliced cups spinach or other greens, such as kale 1 cup sliced berries of your choosing, fresh or frozen
1 orange, peeled and cut into segments
1 cup unsweetened nondairy milk cup ice Directions
In a blender, combine all the Ingredients.

Starting with the blender on low speed, begin blending the smoothie, gradually increasing blender speed until smooth. Serve immediately.

7 Blueberry And Chia Smoothie

Preparation: 10 minutesCooking: 0 minutes Servings: 2
Ingredients

1 tablespoons chia seeds 2 cups unsweetened nondairy milk 2 cups blueberries, fresh or frozen 2 tablespoons pure maple syrup or agave 2 tablespoons cocoa powder

Directions:

Soak the chia seeds in the almond milk for 5 minutes.

In a blender, combine the soaked chia seeds, almond milk, blueberries, maple syrup, and cocoa powder and blend until smooth. Serve immediately.

8. Berries with Mascarpone on Toasted Bread

Preparation Time: 10 minutes Cooking Time: 0 minute
Servings: 1
Ingredients:

1 slice whole-wheat bread

2 tablespoons mascarpone cheese 1/8 cup raspberries 1/8 cup strawberries

1 teaspoon fresh mint leaves Directions:
Spread the cheese on the bread.

Top with the berries and chopped mint leaves. Store in food container and refrigerate.
Toast in the oven when ready to eat.

Nutrition: Calories: 326 fat: 27.3g Saturated fat: 14.2g Cholesterol: 70mg Sodium: 130mg Potassium: 115mg Carbohydrates: 15.1g Fiber: 4.1g Sugar: 3g Protein: 7.9g

9 Fruit Cup

Preparation Time: 15 minutes Cooking Time: 0 minute Servings: 4Ingredients:

2 cups melon, sliced

2 cups strawberries, sliced 2 cups grapes, sliced in half 2 cups peaches, sliced

3 tablespoons freshly squeezed lime juice

½ teaspoon ground ginger1 tablespoon honey
3 teaspoons lime zest

¼ cup coconut flakes, toastedDirections:
Toss the fruits in lime juice, ginger and honey.Sprinkle the lime zest on top.
Top with the coconut flakes.

Nutrition: Calories: 65 Total fat: 1.3g Saturated fat: 1.1g Sodium: 20mg Potassium: 247mg Carbohydrates: 13.9g Fiber: 1.6g Sugar: 10g Protein: 1g

10 Oatmeal with Black Beans & Cheddar

Preparation Time: 10 minutes Cooking Time: 0 minute Servings: 2

Ingredients:

½ cup rolled oats

¼ cup Vegan yogurt

½ cup almond milk

2 tablespoons seasoned black beans

2 tablespoons Cheddar cheese, shredded 1 stalk scallion, minced 1 tablespoon cilantro, chopped

Directions:

Mix all the ingredients except the cilantro in a glass jar with lid. Refrigerate for up to 5 days.

Sprinkle the cilantro on top before serving.

Nutrition: Calories: 47 Total fat: 1.2g Saturated fat: 0.5g Sodium: 30mg Potassium: 151mg Carbohydrates: 11g Fiber: 1.9g Sugar: 9g Protein: 2g

11 Strawberry Smoothie Bowl

Preparation time: 30 minutes Cooking time: 0 minutes
Servings: 02
Ingredients:

Smoothie bowl:

1½ cups frozen strawberries

½ cup coconut milkChia seeds Directions:
In a blender jug, puree all the ingredients for the smooth bowl.Pour the smoothie in the serving bowl.
Add strawberries, banana and chia seeds on top.Chill well then serve.
Nutrition: Calories 275 Total Fat 14.5 g Saturated Fat 12.5 g

Cholesterol 36 mg Sodium 13 mg Total Carbs 25 g Fiber 5 g Sugar 5

g Protein 2.5 g

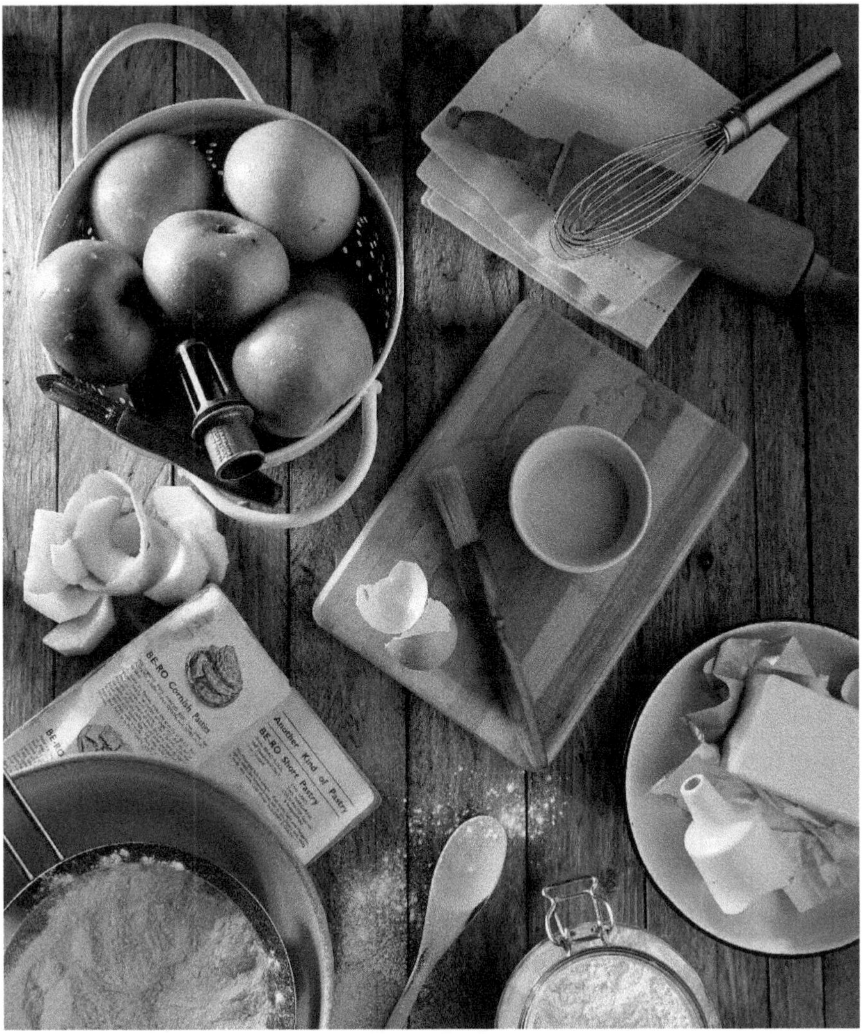
BE-RO Cornish Pasties
Another Kind of Pastry
BE-RO Short Pastry

Soups, Salads, and Sides

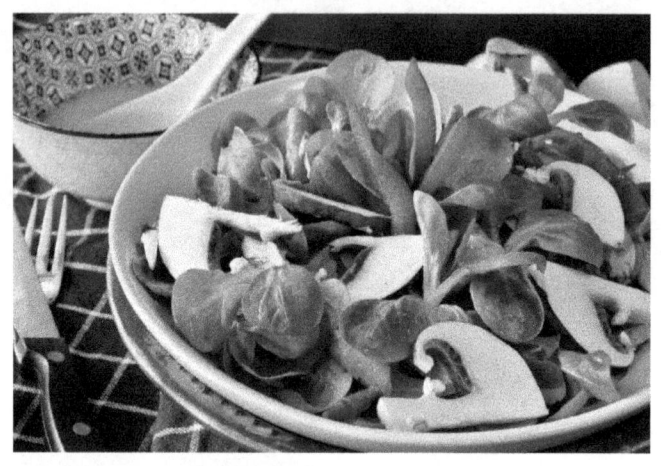

12 Creamy Squash Soup

Preparation time: 35 minutes Cooking time: 22 minutes
Servings: 8
Ingredients:

3 cups butternut squash, chopped

1 ½ cups unsweetened coconut milk1 tbsp coconut oil
1 tsp dried onion flakes1 tbsp curry powder
4 cups water

1 garlic clove

1 tsp kosher saltDirections:
Add squash, coconut oil, onion flakes, curry powder, water, garlic, and salt into a large saucepan. Bring to boil over high heat.

Turn heat to medium and simmer for 20 minutes.

Puree the soup using a blender until smooth. Return soup to the saucepan and stir in coconut milk and cook for 2 minutes.

Stir well and serve hot.

Nutrition: calories 146; fat 12.6 g; carbohydrates 9.4 g; sugar 2.8 g;

protein 1.7 g; cholesterol 0 mg

13 Cucumber Edamame Salad

Preparation time: 5 minutes Cooking time: 8 minutes
Servings: 2
Ingredients:

3 tbsp. Avocado oil

1 cup cucumber, sliced into thin rounds

½ cup fresh sugar snap peas, sliced or whole

½ cup fresh edamame

¼ cup radish, sliced

1 large avocado, peeled, pitted, sliced 1 nori sheet, crumbled

2 tsp. Roasted sesame seeds 1 tsp. Salt
Directions:

Bring a medium-sized pot filled halfway with water to a boil over medium-high heat.

Add the sugar snaps and cook them for about 2 minutes.

Take the pot off the heat, drain the excess water, transfer the sugarsnaps to a medium-sized bowl and set aside for now.

Fill the pot with water again, add the teaspoon of salt and bring to a boil over medium-high heat.

Add the edamame to the pot and let them cook for about

6 minutes.

Take the pot off the heat, drain the excess water, transfer the soybeans to the bowl with sugar snaps and let them cool down for about 5 minutes.

Combine all ingredients, except the nori crumbs and roasted sesameseeds, in a medium-sized bowl.

Carefully stir, using a spoon, until all ingredients are evenly coated in oil. Top the salad with the nori crumbs and roasted sesame seeds.

Transfer the bowl to the fridge and allow the salad to cool for at least30 minutes.

Serve chilled and enjoy!

Nutrition: Calories 409 Carbohydrates 7.1 g Fats 38.25 g Protein 7.6g

14 Best Broccoli Salad

Preparation time: 15 minutes Chilling time: 1 hour
Servings: 8
Ingredients:

8 cups diced broccoli

¼ cup sunflower seeds

3 tablespoons apple cider vinegar

½ cup dried cranberries 1/3 cup cubed onion
1 cup mayonnaise

½ cup bacon bits

2 tablespoons sugar

½ teaspoon salt and ground black pepper Directions:
In a bowl, mix vinegar, salt, pepper, mayonnaise, and sugar. Mix it

well. In another bowl, mix all the remaining ingredients and pour the prepared mayonnaise dressing and mix it well. Before serving to refrigerate it for at least an hour.

Nutrition: Carbohydrates 17g, protein 6g, fats 26g, calories 317

Entrées

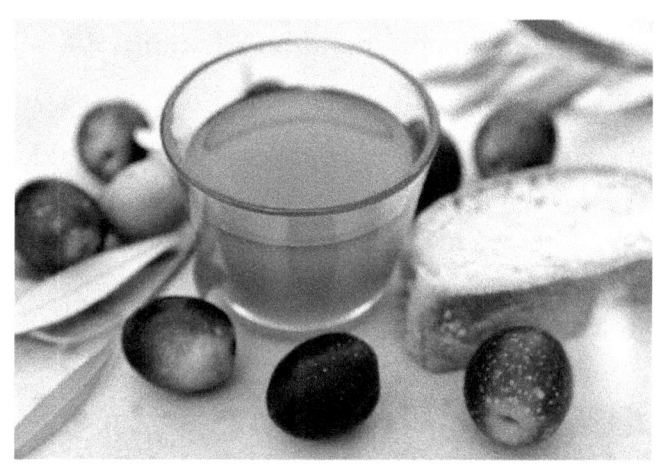

15 Crunchy Asparagus Spears

Preparation time: 25 minutes Cooking time: 25 minutes
Servings: 4
Ingredients:

1 bunch asparagus spears (about 12 spears)

¼ cup nutritional yeast

2 tablespoons hemp seeds 1 teaspoon garlic powder
¼ teaspoon paprika (or more if you like paprika)

⅛ teaspoon ground pepper

¼ cup whole-wheat breadcrumbs Juice of ½ lemon
Directions:

Preheat the oven to 350 degrees, Fahrenheit. Line a Wash the asparagus, snapping off the white part at the bottom. Save it for making vegetable stock.

Mix together the nutritional yeast, hemp seed, garlic powder, paprika, pepper and breadcrumbs.

Place asparagus spears on the baking sheets giving them a little room in between and sprinkle with the mixture in the bowl.

Bake for up to 25 minutes, until crispy.

Serve with lemon juice if desired.

16 Cucumber Bites with Chive and Sunflower Seeds

Preparation time: 5 minutes Cooking time: 5 minutes Servings: 2

Ingredients:

1 cup raw sunflower seed ½ teaspoon salt

½ cup chopped fresh chives 1 clove garlic, chopped

2 tablespoons red onion, minced

2 tablespoons lemon juice

½ cup water (might need more or less) 4 large cucumbers

Directions:

Place the sunflower seeds and salt in the food processor and process to a fine powder. It will take only about 10 seconds.

Add the chives, garlic, onion, lemon juice and water and process until creamy, scraping down the sides frequently. The mixture should be very creamy; if not, add a little more water.

Cut the cucumbers into 1½-inch coin-like pieces.

Spread a spoonful of the sunflower mixture on top and set on a platter. Sprinkle more chopped chives on top and refrigerate until

ready to serve.

Plant Based Diet Recipes 2021

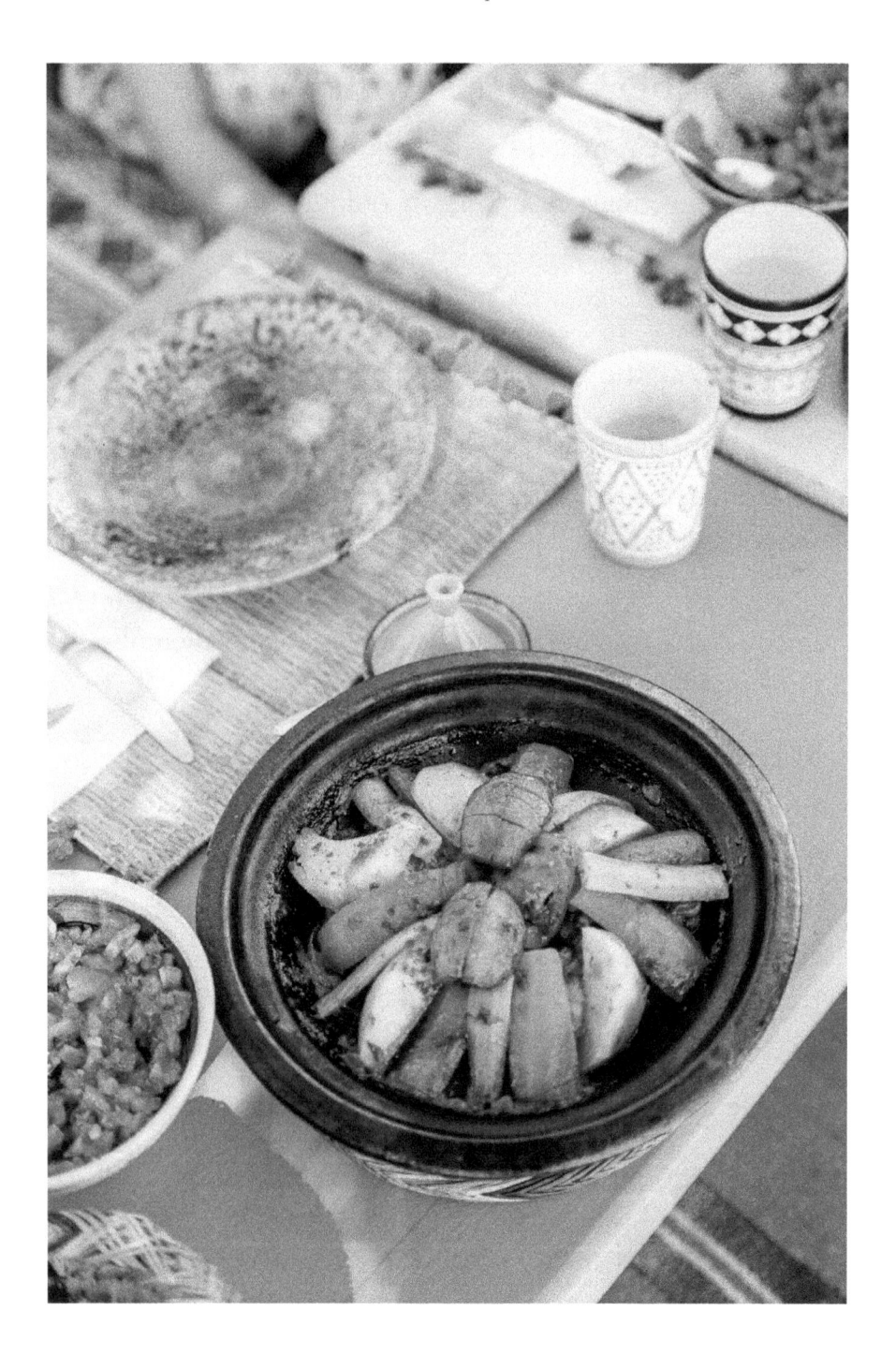

Smoothies and Beverages

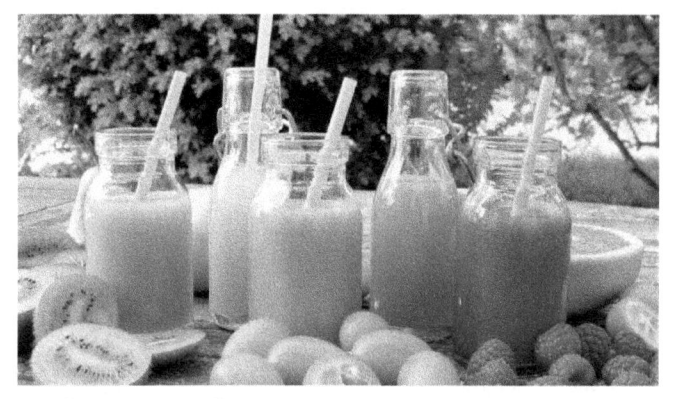

17 Tangy Spiced Cranberry Drink

Preparation time: 3 hours and 10 minutes Cooking time: 3 hours
Servings: 14

Ingredients:

1 1/2 cups of coconut sugar 12 whole cloves

2 fluid ounce of lemon juice

6 fluid ounce of orange juice

32 fluid ounce of cranberry juice 8 cups of hot water
1/2 cup of Red Hot candies

Directions:

Pour the water into a 6-quarts slow cooker along with the cranberry juice, orange juice, and the lemon juice.

Stir the sugar properly.

Wrap the whole cloves in a cheese cloth, tie its corners with strings, and immerse it in the liquid present inside the slow cooker.

Add the red hot candies to the slow cooker and cover it with the lid.

Then plug in the slow cooker and let it cook on the low heat setting for 3 hours or until it is heated thoroughly.

When done, discard the cheesecloth bag and serve.

Nutrition: Calories:89 Cal, Carbohydrates:27g, Protein:0g, Fats:0g, Fiber:1g.

18 Warm Pomegranate Punch

Preparation: 3 hours and 15 minutes Cooking: 3 hours Servings: 10

Ingredients:

3 cinnamon sticks, each about 3 inches long 12 whole cloves
1/2 cup of coconut sugar 1/3 cup of lemon juice

32 fluid ounce of pomegranate juice

32 fluid ounce of apple juice, unsweetened 16 fluid ounce of brewed tea

Directions:

Using a 4-quart slow cooker, pour the lemon juice, pomegranate, juice apple juice, tea, and then sugar.

Wrap the whole cloves and cinnamon stick in a cheese cloth, tie its corners with a string, and immerse it in the liquid present in the slow cooker.

Then cover it with the lid, plug in the slow cooker and let it cook atthe low heat setting for 3 hours or until it is heated thoroughly.

When done, discard the cheesecloth bag and serve it hot or cold.

Nutrition: Calories:253 Cal, Carbohydrates:58g, Protein:7g, Fats:2g,Fiber:3g.

19 Rich Truffle Hot Chocolate

Preparation time: 2 hours and 10 minutes Cooking time: 2 hours
Servings: 4

Ingredients:

1/3 cup of cocoa powder, unsweetened 1/3 cup of coconut sugar 1/8 teaspoon of salt

1/8 teaspoon of ground cinnamon

1 teaspoon of vanilla extract, unsweetened 32 fluid ounce of coconut milk

Directions:

Using a 2 quarts slow cooker, add all the ingredients and stir properly.

Cover it with the lid, then plug in the slow cooker and cook it for 2 hours on the high heat setting or until it is heated thoroughly.

When done, serve right away.

Nutrition: Calories:67 Cal, Carbohydrates:13g, Protein:2g, Fats:2g, Fiber:2.3g.

20 Vanilla Milkshake

Preparation: 5 min.Cooking: 5 min.Servings: 4

Ingredients:

2 c. ice cubes 2 t. vanilla extract

6 tbsp. powdered erythritol1 c. cream of dairy-free

½ c. coconut milkDirections:

In a high-speed blender, add all the ingredients and blend. Add ice cubes and blend until smooth.

Serve immediately and enjoy!

Nutrition: Calories: 125 | Carbohydrates: 6.8 g | Proteins: 1.2 g |Fats: 11.5 g

21 Raspberry Protein Shake

Preparation: 5 min. Cooking: 5 min. Serving: 1 Ingredients: ¼ avocado 1 c. raspberries, frozen 1 scoop protein powder ½ c. almond milk

Ice cubes Directions:

In a high-speed blender add all the ingredients and blend until lumps of fruit disappear.

Add two to four ice cubes and blend to your desired consistency. Serve immediately and enjoy!

Nutrition: Calories: 756 | Carbohydrates: 80.1 g | Proteins: 27.6 g |

Fats: 40.7 g

22 Raspberry Almond Smoothie

Preparation: 5 min.Cooking: 5 min.Serving: 1

Ingredients:

10 Almonds, finely chopped3 tbsp. almond butter
1 c. almond milk 1 c. Raspberries, frozenDirections:
In a high-speed blender, add all the ingredients and blend until

smooth.

Serve immediately and enjoy!

Nutrition: Calories: 449 | Carbohydrates: 26 g | Proteins: 14 g | Fats:35 g

23   Apple Raspberry Cobbler

Preparation Time: 50 minutesServings: 4

A safer type of fruit cobbler where a cut in sugar enhances the fruit.Ingredients

3 apples, peeled, cored, and chopped 2 tbsp pure date sugar cup fresh raspberries

1 tbsp unsalted plant butter

½ cup whole-wheat flour 1 cup toasted rolled oats 2 tbsp pure date sugar 1 tsp cinnamon powderDirections

Preheat the oven to 350 F and grease a baking dish with some plantbutter.

Add the apples, date sugar, and 3 tbsp of water to a medium pot. Cook over low heat until the date sugar melts and then, mix in the raspberries. Cook until the fruits soften, 10 minutes.

Pour and spread the fruit mixture into the baking dish and set aside. In a blender, add the plant butter, flour, oats, date sugar, andcinnamon powder. Pulse a few times until crumbly.

Spoon and spread the mixture on the fruit mix until evenly layered. Bake in the oven for 25 to 30 minutes or until golden brown on top. Remove the dessert, allow cooling for 2 minutes, and serve.

Nutritional info per serving

Calories 539 | Fats 12g| Carbs 105.7g | Protein 8.2g

Snacks and Desserts

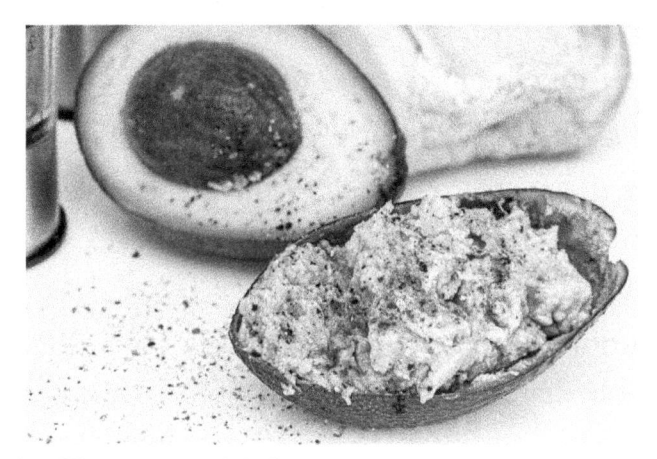

24 Simple Banana Fritters

Preparation time: 15 mins Cooking time: 20 mins Servings: 8

Ingredients
4 Bananas

3 Tbsps. Maple Syrup

¼ Tsp. Cinnamon Powder

¼ Tsp. Nutmeg

1 Cup Coconut Flour

Directions
Preheat oven to 350° F.

Mash the bananas in a large mixing bowl along with maple syrup, cinnamon, nutmeg powder and coconut flour.

Mix all the ingredients well.

Take 2 tbsps. mixture and make small 1-inch-thick

fritters from thismixture.

Place fritters in greased baking tray.

Bake fritters in preheated oven for about 10-15 minutes until goldenfrom both sides.

Once done, take them out of the oven.Serve with coconut cream.
Enjoy!

Nutrition: Protein: 3% 3 kcal Fat: 28% 30 kcal Carbohydrates: 69%

75 kcal

25 Coconut And Blueberries Ice Cream

Preparation time: 5 minsCooking time: 0 mins Servings: 4
Ingredients

1/4 Cup Coconut Cream1 Tbsp. Maple Syrup
¼ Cup Coconut Flour

1 Cup Blueberries

¼ Cup Blueberries For ToppingDirections
Put ingredients into food processor and mix well on high speed.

Pour mixture in silicon molds and freeze in freezer for about 2-4hours.

Once balls are set remove from freezer. Top with berries. Serve cold and enjoy!

Nutrition: Protein: 3% 4 kcal Fat: 40% 60 kcal Carbohydrates: 57%

86 kcal

26 Peach Crockpot Pudding

Preparation time: 15 mins Cooking time: 4 hours Servings: 6

Ingredients

2 Cups Sliced Peaches 1/4 Cup Maple Syrup
1/2 Tsp. Cinnamon Powder

2 Cups Coconut Milk For Serving
½ Cup Coconut Cream 1 Oz. Coconut Flakes Directions
Lightly grease the crockpot and place peaches in the bottom. Add maple syrup, cinnamon powder and milk. Cover and cook on high for 4 hours.

Once cooked remove from crockpot. For serving pour coconut cream.

Top with coconut flakes. Serve and enjoy!

Nutrition: Protein: 3% 11 kcal Fat: 61% 230 kcal Carbohydrates: 36%

133 kcal

27 Green Soy Beans Hummus

Preparation time: 15 minutes Cooking time: 0 minutes
Servings: 6
Ingredients

1 1/2 cups frozen green soybeans 4 cups of water
coarse salt to taste

1/4 cup sesame paste 1/2 tsp grated lemon peel 3 Tbsp fresh lemon juice 2 cloves of garlic crushed 1/2 tsp ground cumin
1/4 tsp ground coriander

4 Tbsp extra virgin olive oil

1 Tbsp fresh parsley leaves chopped

Serving options: sliced cucumber, celery, olives Directions:

1. In a saucepan, bring to boil 4 cups of water with 2 to 3 pinch of coarse salt.

2. Add in frozen soybeans, and cook for 5 minutes or until tender.

3. Rinse and drain soybeans into a colander.

4. Add soybeans and all remaining ingredients into a food processor.

5. Pulse until smooth and creamy.

6. Taste and adjust salt to taste.

7. Serve with sliced cucumber, celery, olives, bread…etc.

28 High Protein Avocado Guacamole

Preparation time: 15 minutes Cooking time: 0 minutes
Servings: 4
Ingredients

1/2 cup of onion, finely chopped

1 chili pepper (peeled and finely chopped) 1 cup tomato, finely chopped Cilantro leaves, fresh 2 avocados

2 Tbsp linseed oil 1/2 cup ground walnuts 1/2 lemon (or lime) Salt

Directions:

Chop the onion, chili pepper, cilantro, and tomato; place in a largebowl.

Slice avocado, open vertically, and remove the pit. Using the spoon take out the avocado flesh.

Mash the avocados with a fork and add into the bowl with onionmixture.

Add all remaining ingredients and stir well until ingredients combinewell.

Taste and adjust salt and lemon/lime juice.

Keep refrigerated into covered glass bowl up to 5 days.

29 Homemade Energy Nut Bars

Preparation time: 15 minutes Cooking time: 0 minutes
Servings: 4
Ingredients

1/2 cup peanuts 1 cup almonds
1/2 cup hazelnut, chopped

1 cup shredded coconut 1 cup almond butter
2 tsp sesame seeds toasted

1/2 cup coconut oil, freshly melted 2 Tbsp organic honey
1/4 tsp cinnamon

Directions

Add all nuts into a food processor and pulse for 1-2 minutes.

Add in shredded coconut, almond butter, sesame seeds, melted coconut oil, cinnamon, and honey; process only for one minute.

Cover a square plate/tray with parchment paper and apply the nut mixture.

Spread mixture vigorously with a spatula. Place in the freezer for 4 hours or overnight.

Remove from the freezer and cut into rectangular bars.

Ready! Enjoy!

30 Chocolate Energy Snack Bar

Preparation Time: 5 MinutesCooking Time: 0 Minutes

Servings: 4Ingredients:

Flax Seeds (1 T.)

Chia Seeds (1 T.) Agave Nectar (2 T.)Almonds (1 C.)

Dried Cranberries (1 C.)Dates (1 C.)

Directions:

When you need a snack that is easy to grab when you are on the go, this is the perfect recipe. You are going to start out by pulsing the almonds and dates in a food processor. Once they are chopped fine, add in the seeds, agave, and cranberries. At this point, pulse until everything is combined.

Next, you will want to add the batter into a lined pan and press everything down into the bottom.

Finally, pop the dish into the fridge for two hours, cut into squares, and your bars are ready!

Nutrition: Calories: 400 Proteins: 10g Carbs: 55g Fats: 20g

31 Zesty Orange Muffins

Preparation Time: 40 Minutes Cooking Time: 20 Minutes
Servings: 11
Ingredients:

Chopped Hazelnuts (3 T.) Orange Juice (1 C.)
Olive Oil (.50 C.)

Baking Powder (2 t.) Brown Sugar (.75 C.) Flour (2 C.)
Baking Soda (1 Pinch) Salt (to Taste)
Orange Zest (2 T.)

Directions:

Muffins are the perfect snack to grab and go when you need to leave the house quickly. Start off by prepping the oven to 350.

As this warms up, take out your mixing bowl and combine the hazelnuts, salt, baking soda, baking powder, sugar, and flour. Once these are mixed together well, add in the olive oil and orange juice.

With your mixture made, evenly pour into lined muffin tins and then pop it into the oven for 20 minutes.

By the end, the muffins should be cooked through and golden at the top. If they look done, remove from the oven, and your snack is ready to go.

Nutrition: Calories: 220 Proteins: 3g Carbs: 30g Fats: 10g

32 Chocolate Tahini Balls

Preparation Time: 10 Minutes Cooking Time: 0 Minutes
Servings: 8
Ingredients:

Sesame Seeds (2 T.)Tahini (2 T.)

Cacao Nibs (2 T.)

Unsweetened Cocoa Powder (2 T.) Old-fashioned Rolled Oats (.25 C.)Medjool Dates (4)
Rock Salt (1 Pinch)Directions:
For this quick snack, start off by placing all of the ingredients aboveinto a blender and blend until you get a dough-like texture.

Next, take the dough and mold it into 8 balls.

Place the balls in the fridge, allow to firm up for 20 minutes, and thenthey will be set.

Nutrition: Calories: 70 Proteins: 2g Carbs: 9g Fats: 4g

Plant Based Diet Recipes 2021

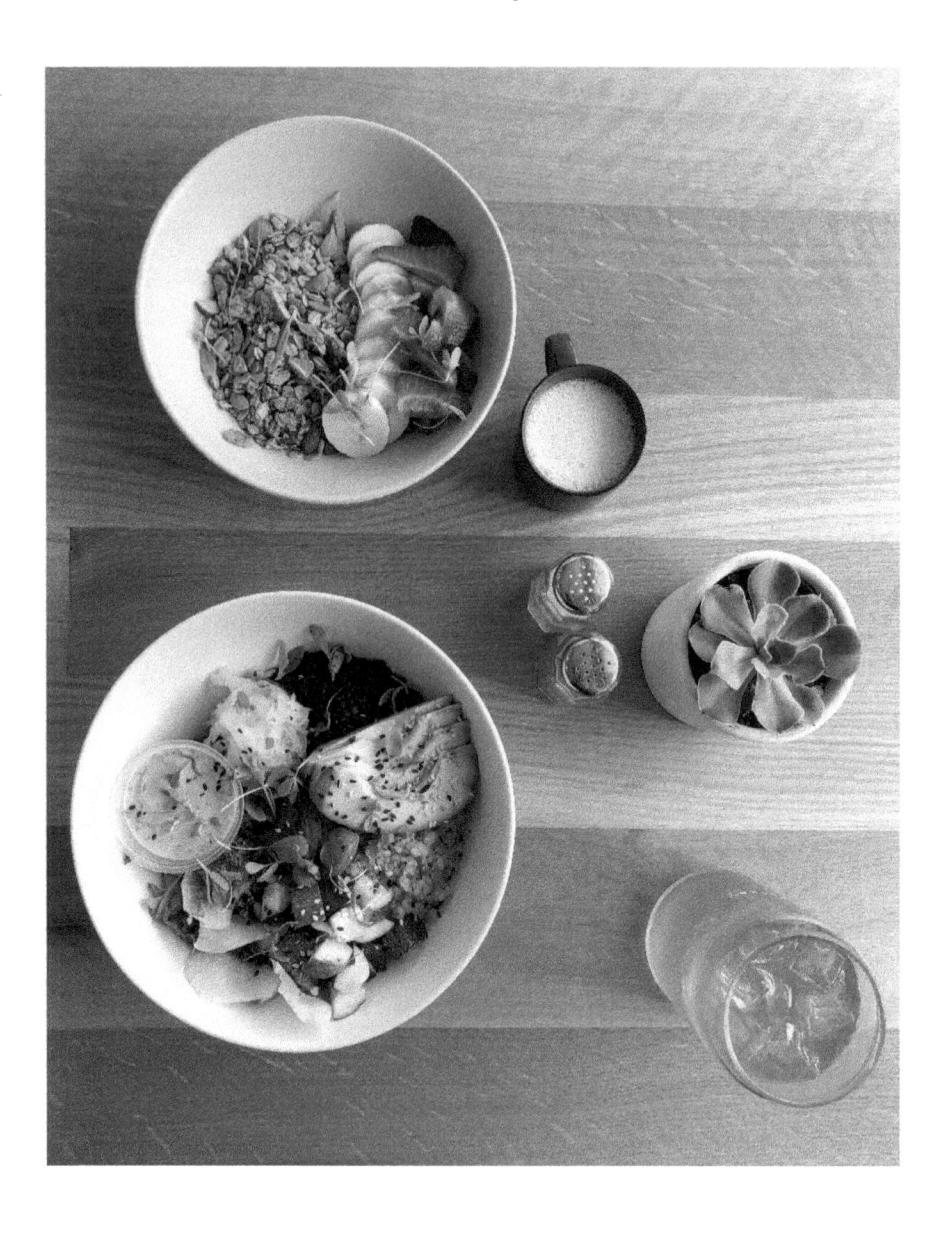

Dinner Recipes

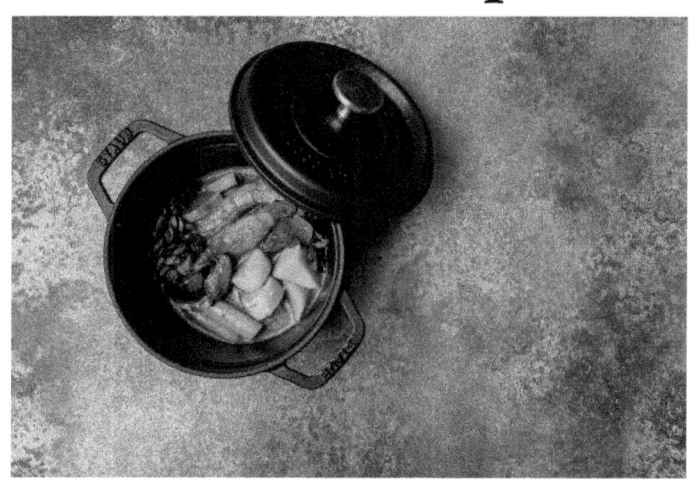

33 Piquillo Salsa Verde Steak

Preparation Time: 30 min. Cooking Time: 25 min. Yields: 8 Servings

Ingredients:

4 – ½ inch thick slices of ciabatta18 oz. firm tofu, drained
5 tbsp. olive oil, extra virgin

Pinch of cayenne

½ t. cumin, ground

1 ½ tbsp. sherry vinegar1 shallot, diced
8 piquillo peppers (can be from a jar) – drained and cut to ½ inchstrips

3 tbsp. of the following:

parsley, finely chopped capers, drained and chopped

Directions:

Place the tofu on a plate to drain the excess liquid, and then sliceinto 8 rectangle pieces.

You can either prepare your grill or use a grill pan. If using a grill pan, preheat the grill pan.

Mix 3 tablespoons of olive oil, cayenne, cumin, vinegar, shallot, parsley, capers, and piquillo peppers in a medium bowl to make our salsa verde. Season to preference with salt and pepper.

Using a paper towel, dry the tofu slices.

Brush olive oil on each side, seasoning with salt and pepper lightly.

Place the bread on the grill and toast for about 2 minutes usingmedium-high heat.

Next, grill the tofu, cooking each side for about 3 minutes or until thetofu is heated through.

Place the toasted bread on the plate then the tofu on top of thebread.

Gently spoon out the salsa verde over the tofu and serve.

Nutrition: Calories: 427 | Carbohydrates: 67.5 g | Proteins: 14.2 g | Fats: 14.6 g

34 Sweet 'n spicy tofu

Preparation time 45 minutes Cooking time: 10 minutes
Servings: 8
Ingredients:

14 ounces extra firm tofu; press the excess liquid and chop intocubes.

3 tablespoons olive oil

2 2-3 cloves garlic, minced

4 tablespoons sriracha sauce or any other hot sauce 2 tablespoons soy sauce
1/4 cup sweet chili sauce

5-6 cups mixed vegetables of your choice (like carrots, cauliflower,broccoli, potato, etc.)

Salt to taste (optional)Direction:
Place a nonstick pan over medium-high heat. Add 1 tablespoon oil.

When oil is hot, add garlic and mixed vegetables and stir-fry until crisp and tender. Remove and keep aside.

Place the pan back on heat. Add 2 tablespoons oil. When oil is hot, add tofu and sauté until golden brown. Add the sautéed vegetables. Mix well and remove from heat.

Make a mixture of sauces by mixing together all the sauces in asmall bowl.

Serve the stir fried vegetables and tofu with sauce.

Lunch Recipes

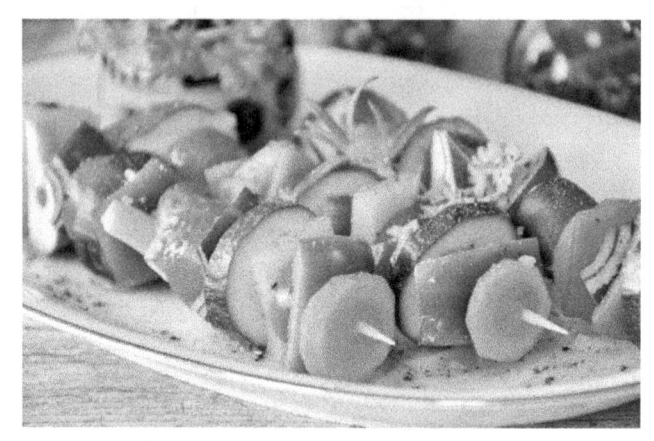

35 Green Pea Fritters

Preparation Time: 10 minutes Cooking Time: 25 minutes
Serving: 4
Ingredients:

For the Fritters:

1 ½ cups (140 grams) chickpea flour 2 cups (250 grams) frozen peas
1 large white onion, peeled, diced

1 tablespoon minced garlic 1/8 teaspoon salt
1 teaspoon baking soda

2 tablespoons mixed dried Italian herbs 1 tablespoon olive oil
Water as needed

For the Yoghurt Sauce:

1/2 teaspoon dried rosemary 1/2 teaspoon dried parsley 1/2 teaspoon dried mint

1 lemon, juiced 1 cup soy yogurtDirections:

Switch on the oven, set it to 350° F and let it preheat.

Take a medium saucepan, place it over medium heat, add peas, cover them with water, bring it to a boil, cook for 2 to 3 minutes until tender, and when done, drain the peas and set aside until required.

Take a frying pan, place it over medium heat, add oil and when hot, add onion and garlic; cook for 5 minutes until softened.

Transfer onion-garlic mixture to a food processor, add peas and pulse for 1 minute until the thick paste comes together.

Tip the mixture in a bowl, add salt, baking soda, Italian herbs, and chickpea flour, stir until incorporated and shape the mixture into ten patties.

Brush the patties with oil, arrange them onto a baking sheet and bake for 15 to 18 minutes until golden brown and thoroughly cooked, turning halfway.

Meanwhile, prepare the yogurt sauce: take a medium bowl, add all the ingredients for it and whisk until combined.

Serve fritters with prepared yogurt sauce.

Nutrition: 94 Cal; 2 g Fat; 0 g Saturated Fat; 14 g Carbs; 3 g Fiber; 4 g Protein; 2 g Sugar

36 Broccoli Rabe

Preparation Time: 15 minutes Cooking Time: 15 minutes
Servings: 8
Ingredients:

2 oranges, sliced in half 1 lb. broccoli rabe
2 tablespoons sesame oil, toasted

Salt and pepper to taste

1 tablespoon sesame seeds, toasted Direction
Pour the oil into a pan over medium heat.

Add the oranges and cook until caramelized. Transfer to a plate.
Put the broccoli in the pan and cook for 8 minutes.
Squeeze the oranges to release juice in a bowl.
Stir in the oil, salt and pepper.

Coat the broccoli rabe with the mixture. Sprinkle seeds on top.
Nutrition: Calories: 59 Total fat: 4.4g   Saturated fat: 0.6g Sodium:

164mg   Potassium: 160mg Carbohydrates: 4.1g Fiber: 1.6g Sugar:2g Protein: 2.2g

37 Whipped Potatoes

Preparation Time: 20 minutes Cooking Time: 35 minutes
Servings: 10
Ingredients:

4 cups water

3 lb. potatoes, sliced into cubes 3 cloves garlic, crushed
6 tablespoons vegan butter 2 bay leaves
10 sage leaves

½ cup Vegan yogurt

¼ cup low-fat milk Salt to taste Direction
Boil the potatoes in water for 30 minutes or until tender. Drain.
In a pan over medium heat, cook the garlic in butter for 1 minute.

Add the sage and cook for 5 more minutes. Discard the garlic.
Use a fork to mash the potatoes.

Whip using an electric mixer while gradually adding the butter, yogurt, and milk.
Season with salt.

Nutrition: Calories: 169 Total fat: 7.6g Saturated fat: 4.7g Cholesterol: 21mg Sodium: 251mg Potassium: 519mg Carbohydrates: 22.1g Fiber: 1.5g Sugar: 2g Protein: 4.2g

38 Chickpea Avocado Sandwich

You can make the chickpea and avocado filling ahead of time and store it in the cold-storage box for or in the icebox. While avocado does brown easily, the lime juice helps preserve the integrity of it.

Preparation time: 10 minutes Cooking Time: 5 minutes Servings: 2

Ingredients: Chickpeas – 1 canAvocado – 1
Dill, dried – .25 teaspoon Onion powder – .25 teaspoon Sea salt – .5 teaspoon Celery, chopped – .25 cup
Green onion, chopped – .25 cup Lime juice – 3 tablespoons Garlic powder – .5 teaspoon Dark pepper, ground – dash Tomato, sliced – 1
Lettuce – 4 leavesBread – 4 slices Directions:

Drain the canned chickpeas and rinse them under cool water. Place them in a bowl along with the herbs, spices, sea salt, avocado, and lime juice. Using a potato masher or fork, mash the avocado and chickpeas together until you have a thick filling. Try not to mash the chickpeas all the way, as they create texture.Stir the celery and green onion into the filling and prepare yoursandwiches.

Layout two slices of bread, top them with the chickpea filling, some lettuce, and sliced tomato. Top them off with the two remainingslices, slice the sandwiches in half, and serve. Nutrition: Calories 471

39 Pizza Bites

Preparation Time: 1 Hour Cooking Time: 30 Minutes
Servings: 4
Ingredients:

Olive Oil (1 t.)

Dried Oregano (1 t.) Lemon Juice (1 t.) Dried Basil (1 t.) Tomato Sauce (1 C.) Cauliflower (1 Head) Salt (to Taste) Nutritional Yeast (to Taste) Garlic Cloves (2, Minced)
Directions:

Begin by prepping the oven to 300 and line a pan with parchment paper. When this is set, take a mixing bowl and combine the olive oil, oregano, basil, salt, tomato sauce, and the basil together. In a second bowl, you will want to place your nutritional yeast.

When you are ready, gently dip the cauliflower pieces into the tomato sauce and then roll in the nutritional yeast. You will want to place these on the baking sheet and continue until all of the cauliflower is covered.

Once the cauliflower is set, place it into the oven for about an hour or until the edges are crispy. Once they are cooked to your liking, remove from the oven and enjoy with some extra sauce for dipping!

Nutrition: Calories: 110 Proteins: 5g Carbs: 17g Fats: 3g

40 Avocado, Spinach and Kale Soup

Preparation time: 10 minutes Cooking time: 0 minutes
Servings: 4
Ingredients:

1 avocados, pitted, peeled and cut in halves 4 cups vegetable stock
2 tablespoons cilantro, chopped

Juice of 1 lime

1 teaspoon rosemary, dried

½ cup spinach leaves

½ cup kale, torn

Salt and black pepper to the tasteDirections:

In a blender, combine the avocados with the stock and the other ingredients, pulse well, divide into bowls and serve for lunch.

Nutrition: calories 300, fat 23, fiber 5, carbs 6, protein 7

41 Curry spinach soup

Preparation: 10 minutesCooking: 0 minutes Servings: 4

Ingredients:

1 cup almond milk

1 tablespoon green curry paste1 pound spinach leaves
1 tablespoon cilantro, chopped

Salt and black pepper to the taste4 cups veggie stock
1 tablespoon cilantro, choppedDirections:

In your blender, combine the almond milk with the curry paste and the other ingredients, pulse well, divide into bowls and serve for lunch. Nutrition: calories 240, fat 4, fiber 2, carbs 6, protein 2

42 Hot roasted peppers cream

Preparation: 10 minutes Cooking: 30 minutesServings: 4
Ingredients:

1 red chili pepper, minced4 garlic cloves, minced

2 pounds mixed bell peppers, roasted, peeled and chopped 4 scallions, chopped1 cup coconut cream
Salt and black pepper to the taste2 tablespoons olive oil
½ tablespoon basil, chopped4 cups vegetable stock
¼ cup chives, chopped

Directions:

Heat up a pot with the oil over medium heat, add the garlic and thechili pepper and sauté for 5 minutes.

Add the peppers and the other ingredients, toss, bring to a simmerand cook over medium heat for 25 minutes.

Blend the soup using an immersion blender, divide into bowls andserve.

Nutrition: calories 140, fat 2, fiber 2, carbs 5, protein 8

Plant Based Diet Recipes 2021

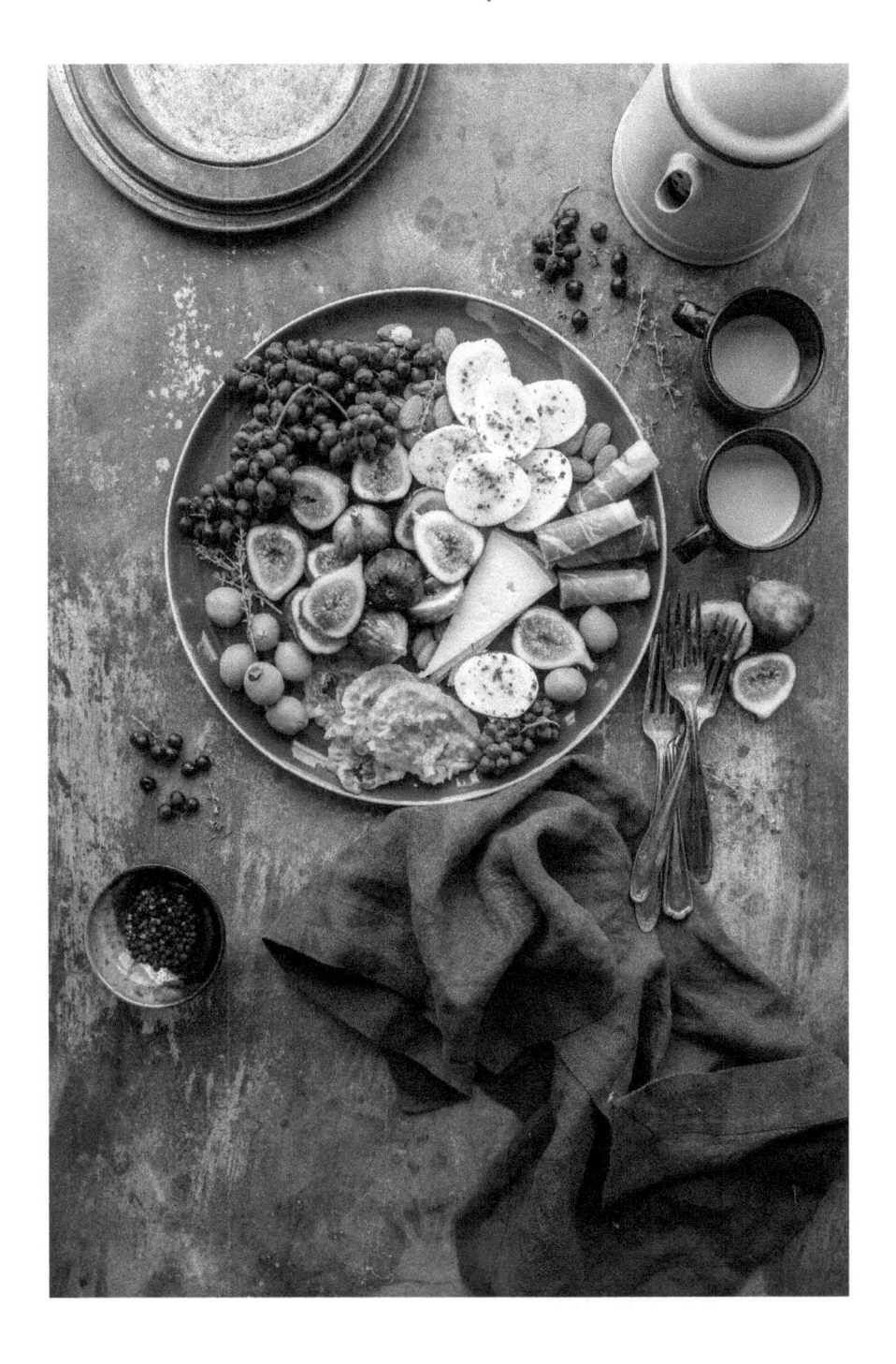

Recipes For Main Courses And Single Dishes

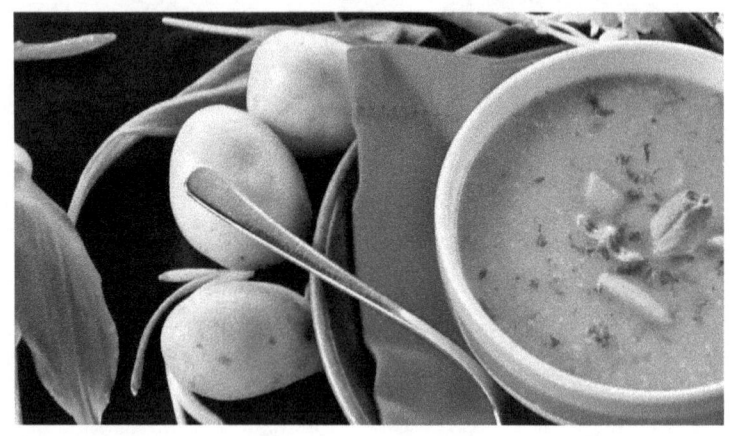

43 Smoked Tempeh with Broccoli Fritters

Preparation Time: 25 minutes Cooking Time: 20 minutes
Servings: 4
Ingredients:

For the flax egg:

4 tbsp flax seed powder + 12 tbsp water For the grilled tempeh:
3 tbsp olive oil

1 tbsp soy sauce

3 tbsp fresh lime juice 1 tbsp grated ginger
Salt and cayenne pepper to taste 10 oz. tempeh slices
For the broccoli fritters:

2 cups of rice broccoli 8 oz. tofu cheese

3 tbsp plain flour

½ tsp onion powder1 tsp salt
¼ tsp freshly ground black pepper4¼ oz. vegan butter

For serving:

½ cup mixed salad greens1 cup vegan mayonnaise
½ lemon, juicedDirections:

For the smoked tempeh:

In a bowl, mix the flax seed powder with water and set aside to soak for 5 minutes.In another bowl, combine the olive oil, soy sauce, lime juice, grated ginger, salt, and cayenne pepper. Brush the tempeh slices with the mixture.

Heat a grill pan over medium heat and grill the tempeh on both sides until nicely smoked and golden brown, 8 minutes. Transfer to a plateand set aside in a warmer for serving.

In a medium bowl, combine the broccoli rice, tofu cheese, flour, onion, salt, and black pepper. Mix in the flax egg until well combine and form 1-inch thick patties out of the mixture.

Melt the vegan butter in a medium skillet over medium heat and fry the patties on both sides until golden brown, 8 minutes. Remove the fritters onto a plate and set aside.

In a small bowl, mix the vegan mayonnaise with the lemon juice.

Divide the smoked tempeh and broccoli fritters onto

serving plates, add the salad greens, and serve with the vegan mayonnaise sauce.

44 Cheesy Potato Casserole

Preparation Time: 30 minutes Cooking Time: 20 minutes
Servings: 4
Ingredients:

2 oz. vegan butter

½ cup celery stalks, finely chopped 1 white onion, finely chopped

1 green bell pepper, seeded and finely chopped Salt and black pepper to taste

2 cups peeled and chopped potatoes 1 cup vegan mayonnaise

4 oz. freshly shredded vegan Parmesan cheese 1 tsp red chili flakes

Directions:

Preheat the oven to 400 F and grease a baking dish with cookingspray.

Season the celery, onion, and bell pepper with salt and blackpepper.

In a bowl, mix the potatoes, vegan mayonnaise, Parmesan cheese,and red chili flakes.

Pour the mixture into the baking dish, add the season vegetables,and mix well.

Bake in the oven until golden brown, about 20 minutes. Remove the baked potato and serve warm with baby spinach.

45 Curry Mushroom Pie

Preparation Time: 65 minutes Cooking Time: 1 hour Servings: 4

Ingredients:

For the piecrust:

1 tbsp flax seed powder + 3 tbsp water

¾ cup plain flour 4 tbsp. chia seeds
4 tbsp almond flour

1 tbsp nutritional yeast 1 tsp baking powder
1 pinch salt

3 tbsp olive oil 4 tbsp water For the filling:
1 cup chopped baby Bella mushrooms 1 cup vegan mayonnaise

3 tbsp + 9 tbsp water

½ red bell pepper, finely chopped 1 tsp curry powder
½ tsp paprika powder ½ tsp garlic powder

¼ tsp black pepper ½ cup coconut cream

1¼ cups shredded vegan Parmesan cheese Directions:
In two separate bowls, mix the different portions of flaxseed powder with the respective quantity of water. Allow soaking for 5 minutes.

For the piecrust:

Preheat the oven to 350 F.

When the flax egg is ready, pour the smaller quantity into a food processor and pour in all the ingredients for the piecrust. Blend until soft, smooth dough forms.

Line an 8-inch springform pan with parchment paper and grease withcooking spray.

Spread the dough in the bottom of the pan and bake for 15 minutes.For the filling:
In a bowl, add the remaining flax egg and all the filling's ingredients.Combine well and pour the mixture on the piecrust. Bake further for 40 minutes or until the pie is golden brown.

Remove from the oven and allow cooling for 1 minute. Slice and serve the pie warm.

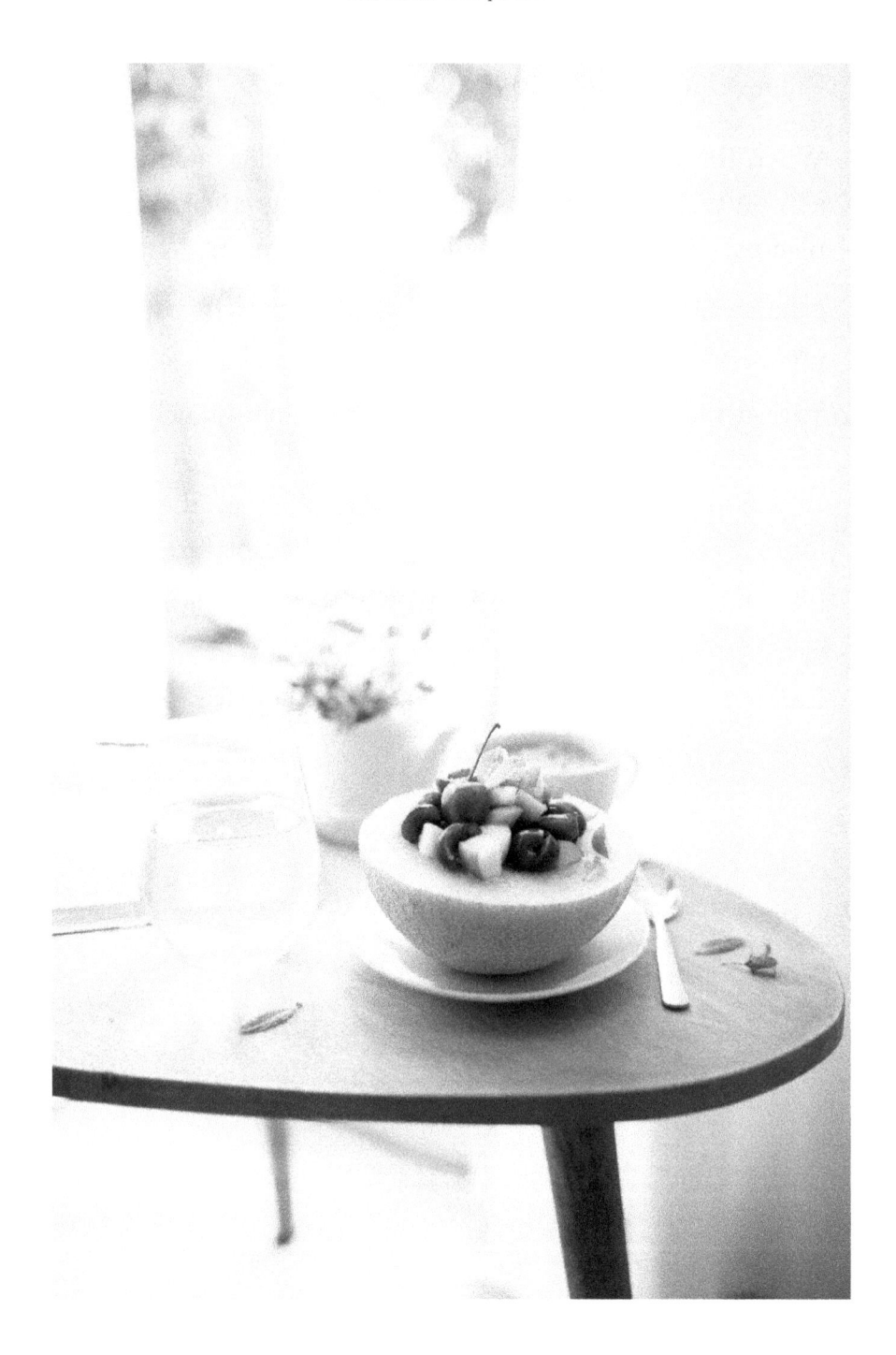

Nutrient-Packed Protein Salads

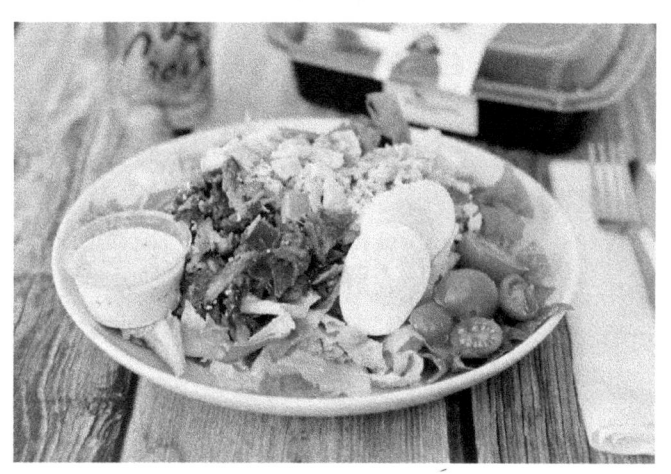

46 Arugula Lentil Salad

Preparation time: 5 mins. Cooking time: 5 mins.

Ingredient: ¾ cups cashews (¾ cups = 100 g) 1 onion

3 tbsp olive oil

1 chilli / jalapeño

5-6 sun-dried tomatoes in oil 3 slices bread (whole wheat)

1 cup brown lentils, cooked (1 cup = 1 / 15oz / 400 g)

1 handful arugula/rocket (1 handful = 100 g) 1-2 tbsp balsamic vinegar

salt and pepper to taste.

Directions:

Roast the cashews on a low heat for about three minutes

in a pan to maximize aroma. Then throw them into the salad bowl. Dice up and fry the onion in one third of the olive oil for about 3 minutes on a low heat. Meanwhile chop the chilli/jalapeño and dried tomatoes. Add them to the pan and fry for another 1-2 minutes. Cut the bread into big croutons. Move the onion mix into a big bowl. Now add the rest of the oil to the pan and fry the chopped-up bread until crunchy. Season with salt and pepper. Wash the arugula and add it to the bowl. Put the lentils in too, and mix them all around. Season with salt, pepper and balsamic vinegar. Serve with the croutons. Super tasty!

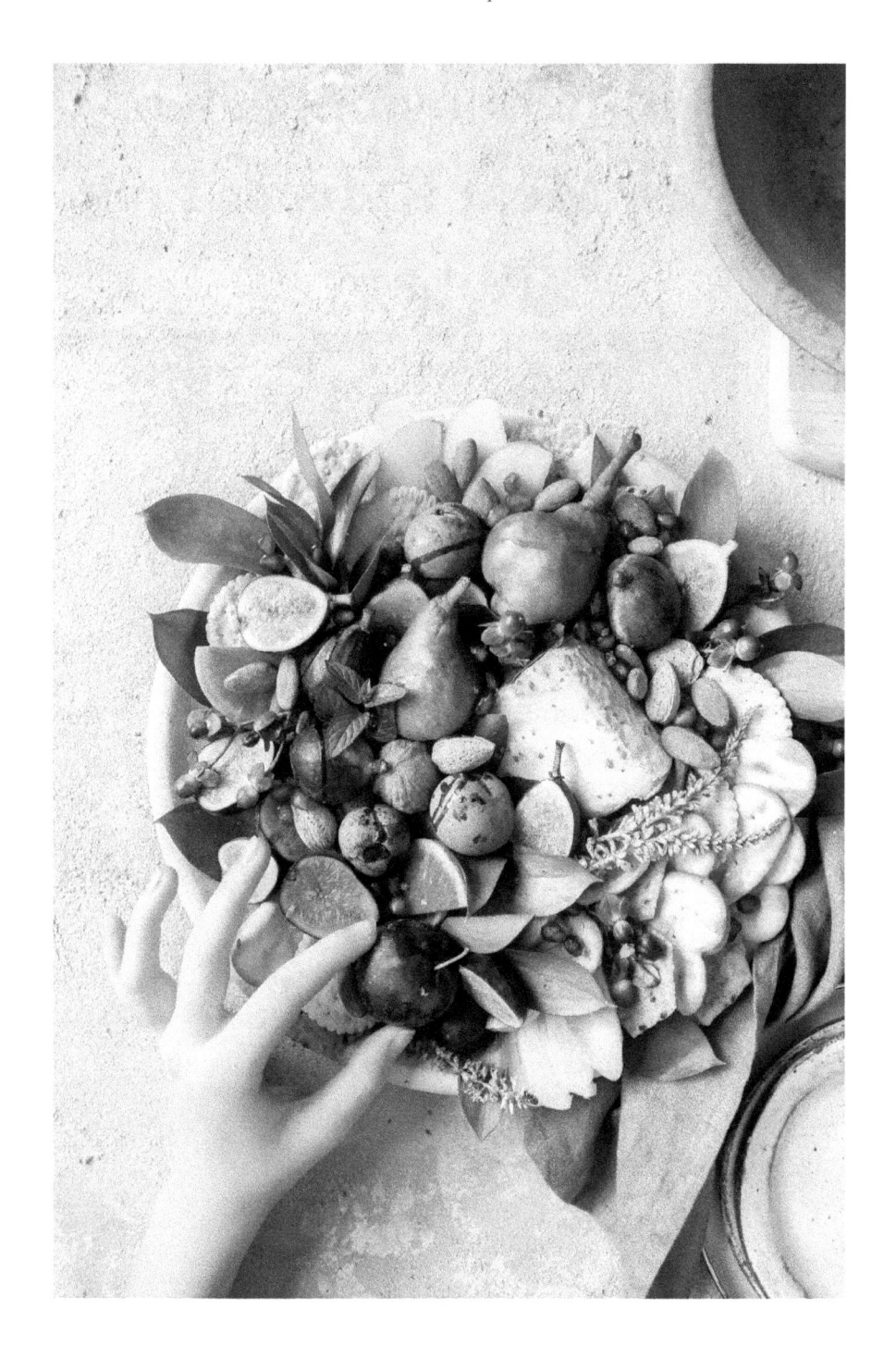

Flavour Boosters (Fish Glazes, Meat Rubs & Fish Rubs)

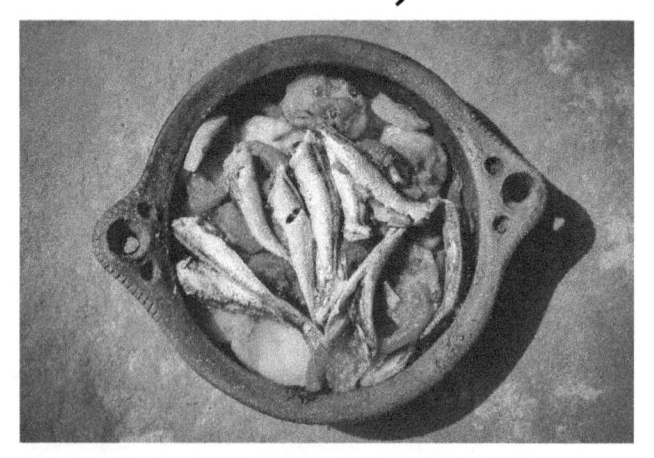

47 Tunisian Mixed Spiced Rub

This incredible rub recipe hailed from the Tunisian cooking secrets; the rub is the essential seasoning base for variety of Tunisian dishes.

This lovely spice blend created by caraway seeds, coriander, and hot pepper works like a charm on your favorite pork tenderloin, chicken as well as salmon.

Preparation Time: 5 min. Cooking Time: 5 min.

Servings: 5-½ tsp. Ingredients:

Coriander seeds - 2 tsp. Caraway seeds - 2 tsp. Crushed red pepper - 3/4 tsp. Garlic powder - 3/4 tsp.

Kosher salt - 1/2 tsp. Directions:

Mix in the coriander seeds, red pepper and caraway seeds

in your spice blender, grinder or processor to make this rub. Start processing or blending the mixed spices on "pulse" mode mixture to ground.

Put the mixed spice mixture into a bowl; mix in the salt and garlic powder. Mix again well.

Now, take your choice of meat cut and place it on a firm surface. Brush or rub the freshly made rub on it; pat gently for the rub to stick onto the surface. Turn the meat cut and repeat to spice up its other side. Repeat with other meat cuts.

The freshly rubbed meat is ready to be grilled or cooked!

48 All Purpose Dill Seed Rub

Boost your steak with vibrant, spiced flavors of this all-purpose dill seed rub. It also beautifully seasons chicken and pork meat cuts. Apply this unique rub minutes before grilling or cooking; you can also store it at room temperature for 12-14 days without sacrificing on its quality.

Preparation Time: 5 min. Cooking Time: 5 min.
Servings: 6-7 tsp.

Ingredients:

Paprika - 2 tsp.

Ground coriander - 2 tsp. Dill seed – 1 tsp.
Dry mustard - ½ tsp. Garlic, minced – 1 clove
Black pepper and salt as required Cayenne pepper - ¼ tsp.
Directions:

Mix in all the rub ingredients in your mixing bowl to make the dillseed rub. Gently mix all ingredients using spatula or spoon to forman aromatic rub mixture.

Now, take your choice of meat cut and place it on a firm surface. Brush the freshly made rub on it; pat gently for the rub to stick onto the surface. Turn the meat cut and repeat to spice up its other side. Repeat with other meat cuts.

Let your meat cuts adequately season for more rich flavors for a few hours in your refrigerator. Take them out, as they are ready to be cooked or grilled!

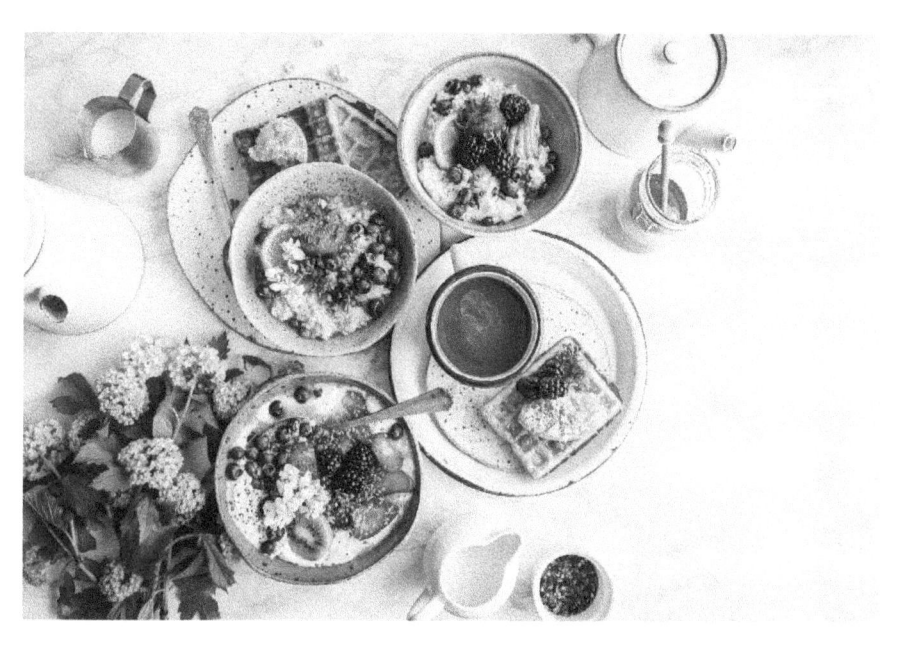

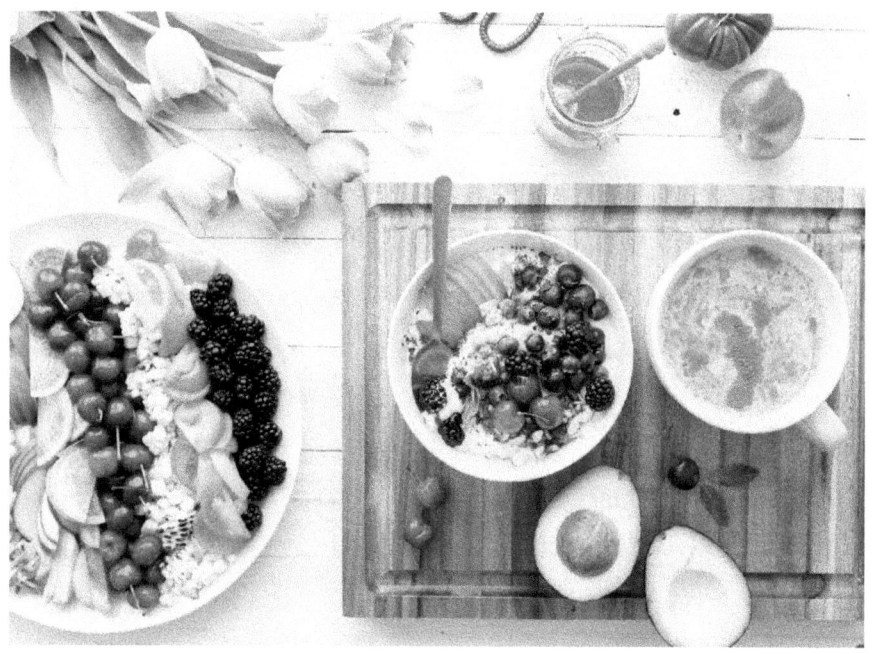

Sauce Recipes

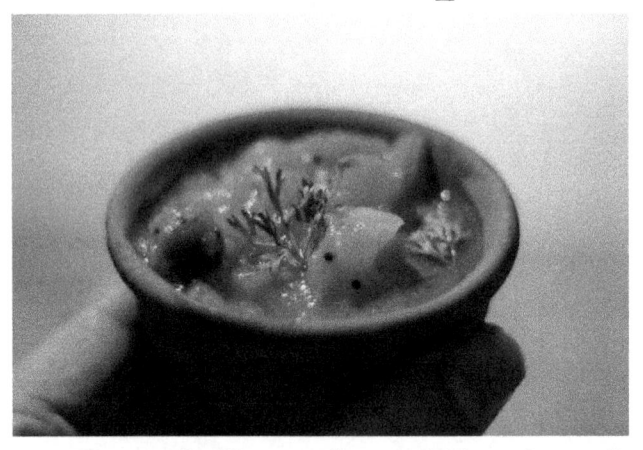

49 Vegan Ranch Dressing (Dipping Sauce)

Preparation time: 5 minutes Cooking time: 5 minutes Servings: 8

Ingredients:

1 tablespoons lemon juice 14 oz. silken tofu
1 tablespoon yellow mustard

1 tablespoon apple cider vinegar 1 teaspoon onion granules
1 tablespoon agave

1 teaspoon garlic granules

2 tablespoons parsley, minced 2 tablespoons dill, minced
1/2 teaspoon Himalayan salt

Directions:

Add all ingredients except parsley and dill to a blender and blend until smooth at high speed.

Add dill and parsley and blend until mixed. Serve chilled.

50 Vegan Smokey Maple BBQ Sauce

Preparation time: 5 minutes Cooking time: 5 minutes
Servings: 8
Ingredients:

1 tablespoon maple syrup 1/2 cup ketchup
1 teaspoon garlic powder 1 teaspoon liquid smoke
Directions:
Add all ingredients to a bowl. Mix them until well combined. Serve and enjoy.

The Complete Plant Based Diet Cookbook

Healthy and Delicious Recipes to Lose Weight Feel Great on a Budget

Frank Smith

Breakfasts

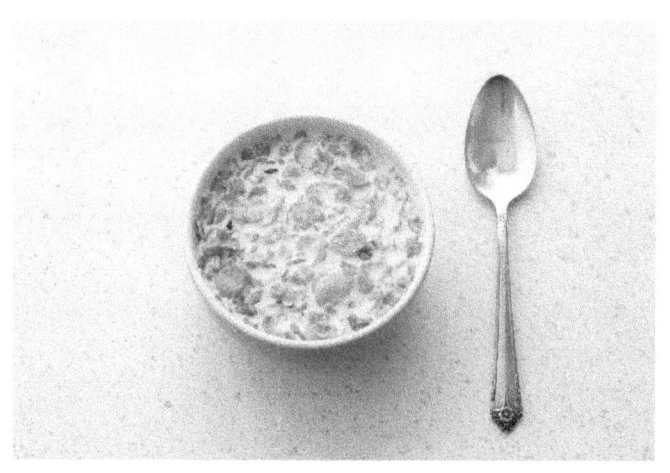

51 Oatmeal Fruit Shake

Preparation Time: 10 minutes Cooking time: 0 minutes
Servings: 2
Ingredients:

1 cup oatmeal, already prepared, cooled 1 apple, cored, roughly chopped
1 banana, halved

1 cup baby spinach 2 cups coconut water 2 cups ice, cubed
½ tsp ground cinnamon 1 tsp pure vanilla extract
Directions:
Add all ingredients to a blender.

Blend from low to high for several minutes until smooth.

Nutrition: Calories 270 Carbohydrates 58 g Fats 1.5 g Protein 5 g

52 Amaranth Banana Breakfast Porridge

Preparation Time: 10 minutes Cooking time: 25 minutes
Servings: 8
Ingredients:

2 cup amaranth

2 cinnamon sticks

4 bananas, diced

2 Tbsp chopped pecans 4 cups water
Directions:

Combine the amaranth, water, and cinnamon sticks, and banana in apot. Cover and let simmer around 25 minutes.

Remove from heat and discard the cinnamon. Places into bowls, andtop with pecans.

Nutrition: Calories 330 Carbohydrates 62 g Fats 6 g Protein 10 g

53 Green Ginger Smoothie

Preparation time: 5 minutes Cooking time: 5 minutes
Servings: 2
Ingredients:

1 banana

½ apple sliced

1 orange sliced and peeled 1 lemon juice

2 big spinach

1 tbsp. fresh ginger

½ cup almond milk

For the dressing: chia seeds, apple, raspberries Directions: Take a blender. Peel off and slice all fruits. Add banana, apple, orange, lime juice, ginger and spinach and blend them well until they turn smooth. Now add almond milk and pulse again for a few seconds. Pour the smoothie into glasses and serve. You can add chia seeds, apple or raspberries for a smoothie bowl. Store it up to 8-10 hours in the refrigerator.

Nutrition: Calories 330 Carbohydrates 62 g Fats 6 g Protein 10 g

54 Chocolate Strawberry Almond Protein Smoothie

Preparation time: 10 mCooking time: 10 m Ingredients:
1 cup of organic strawberries

1 1/2 cup homemade almond milk 1 scoop chocolate protein powder 1 tablespoon organic coconut oil 1/4 cup organic raw almonds

1 tablespoon organic hemp seeds 1 tablespoon organic maca powderFor Garnish:

organic cacao nibs organic hemp seedsDirections:

Put all the ingredients inside a blender and beat until they are wellcombined.

Optional: Garnish with organic hemp seeds or organic cocoa beans.Enjoy it!

Nutrition: carbohydrates: 39 g calories: 720 Fat: 45 g sodium: 732g

protein: 44 g sugar: 12g

55 Apple and Cinnamon Oatmeal

Preparation time: 10 minutes Cooking time: 10 minutes
Servings: 2

Ingredients

1¼ cups apple cider

1 apple, peeled, cored, and chopped

⅔ Cup rolled oats

1 teaspoon ground cinnamon

1 tablespoon pure maple syrup or agave (optional)

Directions

In a medium saucepan, bring the apple cider to a boil over medium-

high heat. Stir in the apple, oats, and cinnamon.

Bring the cereal to a boil and turn down heat to low. Simmer until the oatmeal thickens, 3 to 4 minutes. Spoon into two bowls and sweeten with maple syrup, if using. Serve hot.

56 13 bis. Mango Key Lime Pie Smoothie

Preparation time: 5 minutes Cooking time: 0 minutes Servings: 1

Ingredients

¼ Avocado 1 cup baby spinach

½ Cup frozen mango chunks

1 cup unsweetened soy or almond milk Juice of 1 lime (preferably a key lime). 1 tablespoon maple syrup

Directions

Combine all the Ingredients in a blender and blend until smooth. Enjoy immediately.

57 Spiced Orange Breakfast Couscous

Preparation time: 10 minutes Cooking time: 10 minutes
Servings: 4
Ingredients

3 cups orange juice 1 ½ cups couscous
1 teaspoon ground cinnamon

¼ Teaspoon ground cloves

½ Cup dried fruit, such as raisins or apricots

½ Cup chopped almonds or other nuts or seeds Directions
In a small saucepan, bring the orange juice to a boil. Add the couscous, cinnamon, and cloves and remove from heat. Cover the pan with a lid and allow to sit until the couscous softens, about 5 minutes.

Fluff the couscous with a fork and stir in the dried fruit and nuts. Serve immediately.

58 Fig & Cheese Oatmeal

Preparation Time: 10 minutes Cooking Time: 0 minute Servings: 1

Ingredients:

½ cup water

½ cup rolled oatsPinch salt

2 tablespoons dried figs, sliced

2 tablespoons ricotta cheese

2 teaspoons agave syrup

1 tablespoon almonds, toasted and slicedDirections:

Put the water, oats and salt in a glass jar with lid.Shake to blend well.

Refrigerate for up to 5 days.

Top with the remaining ingredients when ready to serve.

Nutrition: Calories: 294 Total fat: 8.5g Saturated fat: 2.3g Cholesterol: 10mg Sodium: 182mg Potassium: 362mg Carbohydrates: 47.5g Fiber: 6.6g Sugar: 16g Protein: 10.4g

59 Pumpkin Oats

Preparation: 10 minutes Cooking: 0 minute Servings: 1
Ingredients:

½ cup rolle oats ½ cup almond milk ¼ cup ricotta cheese

2 tablespoons pumpkin puree 1 tablespoon maple syrup ¼ teaspoon vanilla 1/8 teaspoon ground nutmeg
Directions:
Combine all the ingredients in a glass jar with lid.

Refrigerate for up to 5 days. Nutrition: Calories: 344 Total fat: 10g Saturated fat: 3.8g Cholesterol: 19mg Sodium: 179mg Potassium: 364mg Carbohydrates: 51.7g Fiber: 5.7g Sugar: 16g Protein: 13.3g

60 Apple Chia Pudding

Preparation time: 10 minutes Cooking time: 5 minutes
Servings: 04
Ingredients:

Chia Pudding:

4 tablespoons chia seeds 1 cup almond milk
½ teaspoon cinnamon Apple Pie Filling:

1 large apple, peeled, cored and chopped

¼ cup water

2 teaspoons maple syrup Pinch cinnamon
2 tablespoons golden raisins Directions:
In a sealable container, add cinnamon, chia seeds and almond milk,

mix well.

Seal the container and refrigerate overnight.

In a medium pot, combine all apple pie filling ingredients and cook for 5 minutes.

Serve the chia pudding with apple filling on top. Enjoy.
Nutrition: Calories 387 Total Fat 5.8g Saturated Fat 4.2 g

Cholesterol 41 mg Sodium 154 mg Total Carbs 24.1 g Fiber 2.9 g

Sugar 3.1 g Protein 6.6 g

Soups, Salads, and Sides

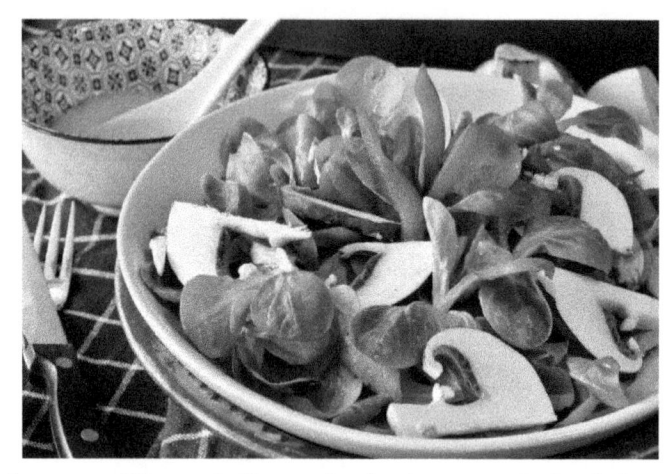

61 Garden Patch Sandwiches on Multigrain Bread

Preparation time: 15 minutes Cooking time: 0 minutes Servings: 4 sandwiches Ingredients:

1 pound extra-firm tofu, drained and patted dry 1 medium red bell pepper, finely chopped

1 celery rib, finely chopped

3 green onions, minced

¼ cup shelled sunflower seeds

½ cup vegan mayonnaise, homemade or store-bought

½ teaspoon salt

½ teaspoon celery salt

¼ teaspoon freshly ground black pepper 8 slices whole grain

bread

4 (¼-inch) slices ripe tomato

4 lettuce leavesDirections:

Crumble the tofu and place it in a large bowl. Add the bell pepper, celery, green onions, and sunflower seeds. Stir in the mayonnaise, salt, celery salt, and pepper and mix until well combined.

Toast the bread, if desired. Spread the mixture evenly onto 4 slices of the bread. Top each with a tomato slice, lettuce leaf, and the remaining bread. Cut the sandwiches diagonally in half and serve.

62 Garden Salad Wraps

Preparation time: 15 minutes Cooking time: 10 minutes Servings: 4 wraps Ingredients:

6 tablespoons olive oil

1-pound extra-firm tofu, drained, patted dry, and cut into ½-inch strips

1 tablespoon soy sauce

¼ cup apple cider vinegar

1 teaspoon yellow or spicy brown mustard

½ teaspoon salt

¼ teaspoon freshly ground black pepper 3 cups shredded romaine lettuce

3 ripe roma tomatoes, finely chopped

1 large carrot, shredded

1 medium english cucumber, peeled and chopped

⅓ cup minced red onion

¼ cup sliced pitted green olives

4 (10-inch) whole-grain flour tortillas or lavash flatbread Directions:

In a large skillet, heat 2 tablespoons of the oil over medium heat. Add the tofu and cook until golden brown, about 10 minutes. Sprinkle with soy sauce and set aside to cool.

In a small bowl, combine the vinegar, mustard, salt, and pepper with the remaining 4 tablespoons oil, stirring to blend well. Set aside.

In a large bowl, combine the lettuce, tomatoes, carrot, cucumber, onion, and olives. Pour on the dressing and toss to coat.

To assemble wraps, place 1 tortilla on a work surface and spread with about one-quarter of the salad. Place a few strips of tofu on the tortilla and roll up tightly. Slice in half

63 Marinated Mushroom Wraps

Preparation time: 15 minutes Cooking time: 0 minutes Servings: 2 wraps Ingredients:

3 tablespoons soy sauce

3 tablespoons fresh lemon juice

1 1/2 tablespoons toasted sesame oil

2 portobello mushroom caps, cut into ¼-inch strips 1 ripe hass avocado, pitted and peeled
2 cups fresh baby spinach leaves

1 medium red bell pepper, cut into ¼-inch strips 1 ripe tomato, chopped
Salt and freshly ground black pepper

Directions:

In a medium bowl, combine the soy sauce, 2 tablespoons of the lemon juice, and the oil. Add the portobello strips, toss to combine, and marinate for 1 hour or overnight. Drain the mushrooms and set aside.

Mash the avocado with the remaining 1 tablespoon of lemon juice.

To assemble wraps, place 1 tortilla on a work surface and spread with some of the mashed avocado. Top with a layer of baby spinach leaves. In the lower third of each tortilla, arrange strips of the soakedmushrooms and some of the bell pepper strips. Sprinkle with the tomato and salt and black pepper to taste. Roll up tightly and cut in half diagonally. Repeat with the remaining ingredients and serve.

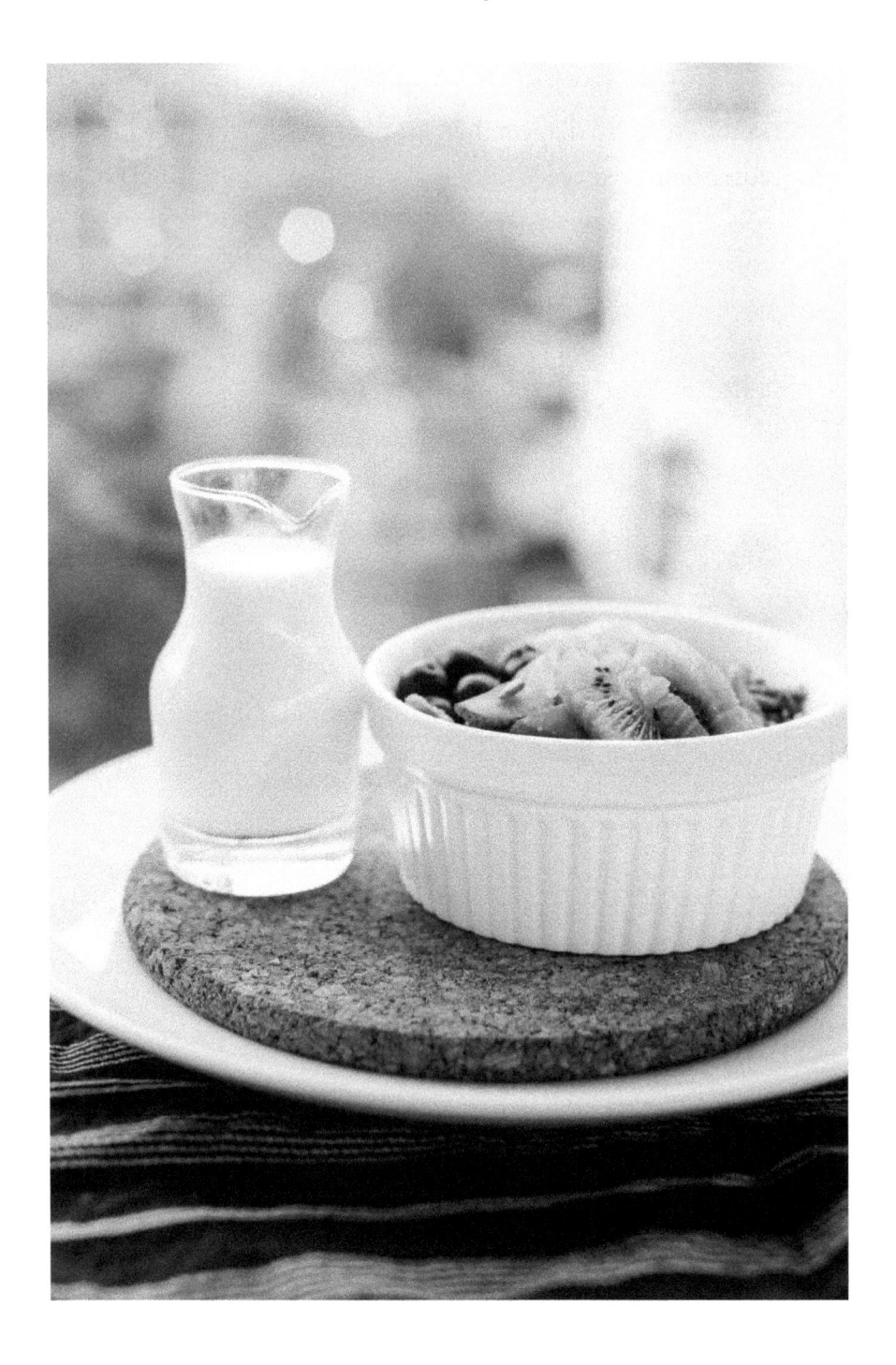

Entrées

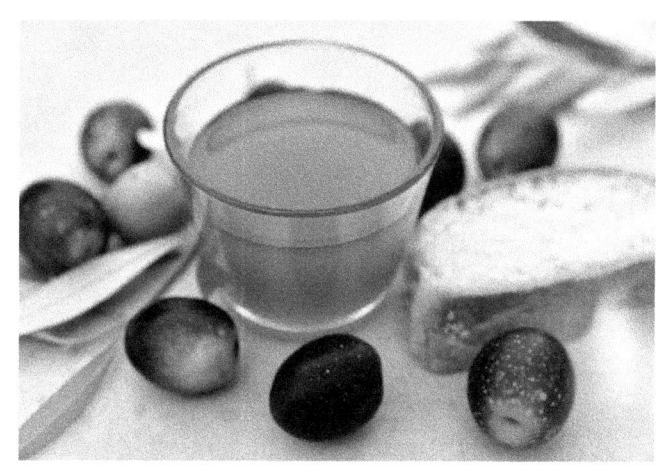

64 Homemade Trail Mix

Preparation time: 20 minutes Cooking time: 20 minutes Servings: 2

Ingredients:

½ cup uncooked old-fashioned oatmeal

½ cup chopped dates

2 cups whole grain cereal

¼ cup raisins

¼ cup almonds

¼ cup walnutsDirections:

Mix all the ingredients in a large bowl.

Place in an airtight container until ready to use.

65 Nut Butter Maple Dip

Preparation time: 1 hourCooking time: 1 hour Servings: Ingredients:

½ tablespoon ground flaxseed 1 teaspoon ground cinnamon

½ tablespoon maple syrup

2 tablespoons cashew milk

¾ cups crunchy, unsweetened peanut butterDirections:

In a bowl, combine the flaxseed, cinnamon, maple syrup, cashew

milk and peanut butter.

Use a fork to mix everything in. I stir it like I'm scrambling eggs. Themixture should be creamy. If it's too runny, add a little more peanut butter; if it's too thick, add a little more cashew milk.

Refrigerate for about an hour, covered and serve.

Smoothies and Beverages

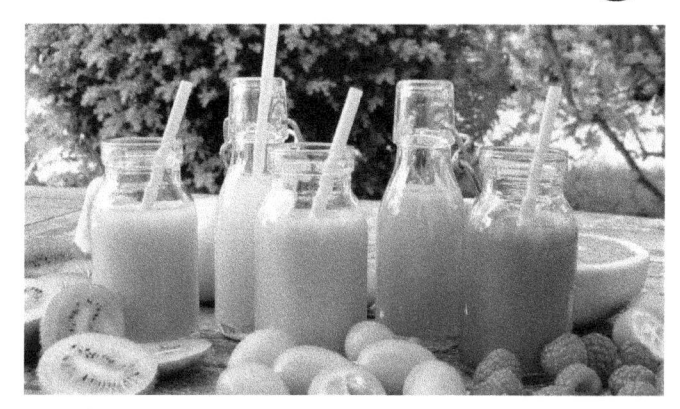

66 Kale & Avocado Smoothie

Preparation Time: 10 Minutes Cooking time: 0 minute Servings: 1

Ingredients:

1 ripe banana

1 cup kale

1 cup almond milk

¼ avocado

1 tbsp. chia seeds 2 tsp. honey
1 cup ice cubes

Direction:

Blend all the ingredients until smooth.

Nutrition: Calories 343 Total Fat 14 gSaturated Fat 2 g Cholesterol 0 mgSodium 199 mgTotal Carbohydrate

55 g Dietary Fiber 12 g Protein 6 gTotal Sugars 29 gPotassium 1051mg

67 Coconut & Strawberry Smoothie

Preparation Time: 10 Minutes Cooking Time: 0 minutes
Serves: 1
Calories: 278

Protein: 14 Grams

Fat: 2 Grams

Carbs: 57 GramsIngredients:
1 Cup Strawberries, Frozen & Thawed Slightly

1 Ripe Banana, Sliced & Frozen

½ Cup Coconut Milk, Light

½ Cup Vegan Yogurt

1 Tablespoon Chia Seeds

1 Teaspoon Lime juice, Fresh4 Ice Cubes
Directions:

Blend everything together until smooth, and serve immediately.

68 Pumpkin Chia Smoothie

Preparation Time: 5 Minutes Cooking Time: 0 minutes
Serves: 1
Calories: 726

Protein: 5.5 Grams

Fat: 69.8 Grams

Carbs: 15 GramsIngredients:
3 Tablespoons Pumpkin Puree

1 Tablespoon MCT Oil

¾ Cup Coconut Milk, Full Fat

½ Avocado, Fresh

1 Teaspoon Vanilla, Pure

½ Teaspoon Pumpkin Pie SpiceDirections:
Combine all ingredients together until blended.

69 Mini Berry Tarts

Preparation Time: 35 minutes + 1 hour chilling Servings: 4 Tickle-sized berries-filled with surprises, oh so delicious! Also so delicious that you can't stop having them.

Ingredients

For the piecrust:

4 tbsp flax seed powder + 12 tbsp water

1/3 cup whole-wheat flour + more for dusting

½ tsp salt

¼ cup plant butter, cold and crumbled 3 tbsp pure malt syrup
1 ½ tsp vanilla extract For the filling:
6 oz cashew cream

6 tbsp pure date sugar

¾ tsp vanilla extract

1 cup mixed frozen berries Directions
Preheat the oven to 350 F and grease a mini pie pans with cooking

spray.

In a medium bowl, mix the flax seed powder with water and allow soaking for 5 minutes.

In a large bowl, combine the flour and salt. Add the

butter and using an electric hand mixer, whisk until crumbly. Pour in the flax egg, malt

syrup, vanilla, and mix until smooth dough forms.

Flatten the dough on a flat surface, cover with plastic wrap, and refrigerate for 1 hour.

After, lightly dust a working surface with some flour, remove the dough onto the surface, and using a rolling pin, flatten the dough intoa 1-inch diameter circle,

Use a large cookie cutter, cut out rounds of the dough and fit into the pie pans. Use a knife to trim the edges of the pan. Lay a parchment paper on the dough cups, pour on some baking beans and bake in the oven until golden brown, 15 to 20 minutes.

Remove the pans from the oven, pour out the baking beans, and allow cooling.

In a medium bowl, mix the cashew cream, date sugar, and vanilla extract.

Divide the mixture into the tart cups and top with berries. Serve immediately.

Nutritional info per serving

Calories 545 | Fats 33.5g| Carbs 53.6g | Protein 10.6g

70 Mixed Nut Chocolate Fudge

Preparation Time: 2 hours 10 minutes

Servings: 4

A recipe for chocolate fudge that takes just 10 minutes to make andrequires ingredients that are readily available.

Ingredients

3 cups unsweetened chocolate chips

¼ cup thick coconut milk

1 ½ tsp vanilla extractA pinch salt
1 cup chopped mixed nuts

Directions

Line a 9-inch square pan with baking paper and set aside.

Melt the chocolate chips, coconut milk, and vanilla in a medium potover low heat.

Mix in the salt and nuts until well distributed and pour the mixtureinto the square pan.

Refrigerate for at least for at least 2 hours.

Remove from the fridge, cut into squares and serve.
Nutritional info per serving
Calories 907 | Fats 31.5g| Carbs 152.1g | Protein 7.7g

71 Date Cake Slices

Preparation Time: 1 hour 20 minutes

Servings: 4

With a slightly thick yet fluffy texture, they're super soft.
Ingredients

½ cup cold plant butter, cut in pieces, plus extra for greasing1 tbsp flax seed powder + 3 tbsp water
½ cup whole-wheat flour, plus extra for dusting

¼ cup chopped pecans and walnuts1 tsp baking powder
1 tsp baking soda

1 tsp cinnamon powder

1 tsp salt

1/3 cup water

1/3 cup pitted dates, chopped

½ cup pure date sugar1 tsp vanilla extract
¼ cup pure date syrup for drizzling.

Directions

Preheat the oven to 350 F and lightly grease a round baking dishwith some plant butter.

In a small bowl, mix the flax seed powder with water and allow thickening for 5 minutes to make the flax egg.

In a food processor, add the flour, nuts, baking powder, baking soda, cinnamon powder, and salt. Blend until well combined.

Add the water, dates, date sugar, and vanilla. Process until smooth with tiny pieces of dates evident.

Pour the batter into the baking dish and bake in the oven for 1 hour and 10 minutes or until a toothpick inserted comes out clean. Remove the dish from the oven, invert the cake onto a serving platter to cool, drizzle with the date syrup, slice, and serve.

Nutritional info per serving

Calories 850 | Fats 61.2g | Carbs 65.7g | Protein 12.8g

72 Chocolate Mousse Cake

Preparation Time: 40 minutes + 6 hours 30 minutes chillingServings: 4

Have a cake with a basic mousse of chocolate and tell me how youfeel.

Ingredients

2/3 cup toasted almond flour

¼ cup unsalted plant butter, melted

2 cups unsweetened chocolate bars, broken into pieces 2 ½ cups coconut cream

Fresh raspberries or strawberries for toppingDirections

Lightly grease a 9-inch springform pan with some plant butter andset aside.

Mix the almond flour and plant butter in a medium bowl and pour the mixture into the springform pan. Use the spoon to spread and press the mixture into the bottom of the pan. Place in the refrigerator to firm for 30 minutes.

Meanwhile, pour the chocolate in a safe microwave bowl and meltfor 1 minute stirring every 30 seconds.

Remove from the microwave and mix in the coconut cream and maple syrup.

Remove the cake pan from the oven, pour the chocolate mixture on top making to sure to shake the pan and even the layer. Chill further for 4 to 6 hours.

Take out the pan from the fridge, release the cake and garnish with the raspberries or strawberries.

Slice and serve. Nutritional info per serving

Calories 608 | Fats 60.5g | Carbs 19.8g | Protein 6.3g

Snacks and Desserts

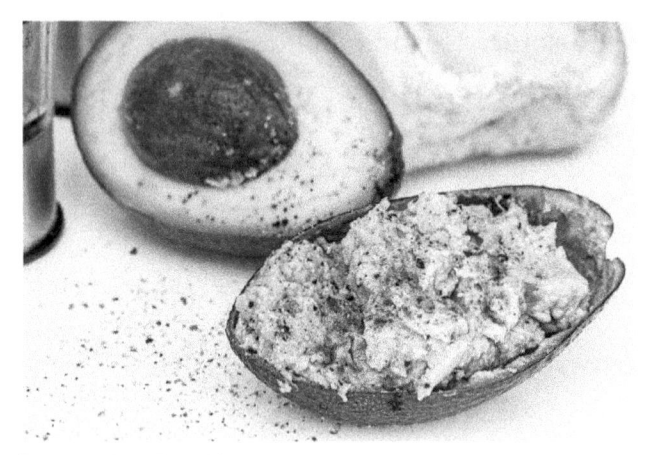

73 Nori Snack Rolls

Preparation Time: 5 minutes Cooking time: 10 minutes
Servings: 4 rolls
Ingredients

2 tablespoons almond, cashew, peanut, or others nut butter2 tablespoons tamari, or soy sauce
4 standard nori sheets

1 mushroom, sliced

1 tablespoon pickled ginger

½ cup grated carrotsDirections
Preparing the Ingredients. Preheat the oven to 350°F.
Mix together the nut butter and tamari until smooth and very thick. Lay out a nori sheet, rough side up, the long way.

Spread a thin line of the tamari mixture on the far end of

the nori sheet, from side to side. Lay the mushroom slices, ginger, and carrots in a line at the other end (the end closest to you).

Fold the vegetables inside the nori, rolling toward the tahini mixture, which will seal the roll. Repeat to make 4 rolls.

Put on a baking sheet and bake for 8 to 10 minutes, or until the rolls are slightly browned and crispy at the ends. Let the rolls cool for a few minutes, then slice each roll into 3 smaller pieces.

Nutrition: Calories: 79; Total fat: 5g; Carbs: 6g; Fiber: 2g; Protein: 4g

74 Risotto Bites

Preparation Time: 15 minutes Cooking time: 20 minutes Servings: 12 bites Ingredients
½ cup panko bread crumbs 1 teaspoon paprika
1 teaspoon chipotle powder or ground cayenne pepper

1½ cups cold Green Pea Risotto Nonstick cooking spray
Directions
Preparing the Ingredients. Preheat the oven to 425°F. Line a baking sheet with parchment paper.

On a large plate, combine the panko, paprika, and chipotle powder. Set aside.

Roll 2 tablespoons of the risotto into a ball.

Gently roll in the bread crumbs, and place on the prepared baking sheet. Repeat to make a total of 12 balls.

Spritz the tops of the risotto bites with nonstick cooking spray and bake for 15 to 20 minutes, until they begin to brown. Cool completely before storing in a large airtight container in a single layer (add a piece of parchment paper for a second layer) or in a plastic freezer bag.

Nutrition: Calories: 100; Fat: 2g; Protein: 6g; Carbohydrates: 17g; Fiber: 5g; Sugar: 2g; Sodium: 165 mg

75 Jicama and Guacamole

Preparation Time: 15 minutes Cooking time: 0 minutes
Servings: 4

Ingredients

juice of 1 lime, or 1 tablespoon prepared lime juice

2 hass avocados, peeled, pits removed, and cut into cubes

½ teaspoon sea salt

½ red onion, minced 1 garlic clove, minced
¼ cup chopped cilantro (optional)

1 jicama bulb, peeled and cut into matchsticksDirections Preparing the Ingredients.

In a medium bowl, squeeze the lime juice over the top of theavocado and sprinkle with salt.

Lightly mash the avocado with a fork. Stir in the onion, garlic, andcilantro, if using.

Serve with slices of jicama to dip in guacamole.

To store, place plastic wrap over the bowl of guacamole andrefrigerate. The guacamole will keep for about 2 days.

76 Oven-baked Caramelize Plantains

Preparation time: 30 minutes Cooking time: 17 minutes
Servings: 4
Ingredients

4 medium plantains, peeled and sliced2 Tbsp fresh orange juice

4 Tbsp brown sugar or to taste

1 Tbsp grated orange zest

4 Tbsp coconut butter, meltedDirections
Preheat oven to 360 F/180 C.

Place plantain slices in a heatproof dish.

Pour the orange juice over plantains, and then sprinkle with brownsugar and grated orange zest.

Melt coconut butter and pour evenly over plantains. Cover with foil and bake for 15 to 17 minutes.
Serve warm or cold with honey or maple syrup.

77 Powerful Peas & Lentils Dip

Preparation time: 10 minutes Cooking time: 0 minutes
Servings: 4
Ingredients

4 cups frozen peas

2 cup green lentils cooked 1 piece of grated ginger
1/2 cup fresh basil chopped 1 cup ground almonds Juice of 1/2 lime
Pinch of salt

4 Tbsp sesame oil

1/4 cup Sesame seeds Directions
Place all ingredients in a food processor or in a blender.

Blend until all ingredients combined well.

Keep refrigerated in an airtight container up to 4 days.

78 Protein "Raffaello" Candies

Preparation time: 15 minutes Cooking time: 0 minutes
Servings: 12

Ingredients

1 1/2 cups desiccated coconut flakes 1/2 cup coconut butter softened
4 Tbsp coconut milk canned

4 Tbs coconut palm sugar (or granulated sugar) 1 tsp pure vanilla extract1 Tbsp vegan protein powder (pea or soy) 15 whole almonds

Directions

Put 1 cup of desiccated coconut flakes, and all remaining ingredients in the blender (except almonds), and blend until soft.

If your dough is too thick, add some coconut milk. In a bowl, add remaining coconut flakes.

Coat every almond in one tablespoon of mixture and roll into a ball. Roll each ball in coconut flakes.

Chill in the fridge for several hours.

79 Roasted Cauliflower

Preparation Time: 30 Minutes Cooking Time: 20 Minutes Servings: 4

Ingredients:

Olive Oil (1 T.) Cauliflower (1, Chopped) Salt (to Taste)

Smoked Paprika (2 t.) Parsley (2 T.) Directions:

If you like to snack, it is better to have healthier options at hand. You'll want to start this recipe off by prepping your oven to 450.

As this warms up, place the cauliflower florets into a large mixing bowl and toss with the olive oil, salt, and smoked paprika. Once this is complete, lay it across a baking sheet and pop it into the oven for 20 minutes.

When the cauliflower is cooked to your liking, remove from the oven, top with parsley, and you are all set.

Nutrition: Calories: 70 Proteins: 3g Carbs: 8g Fats: 5g

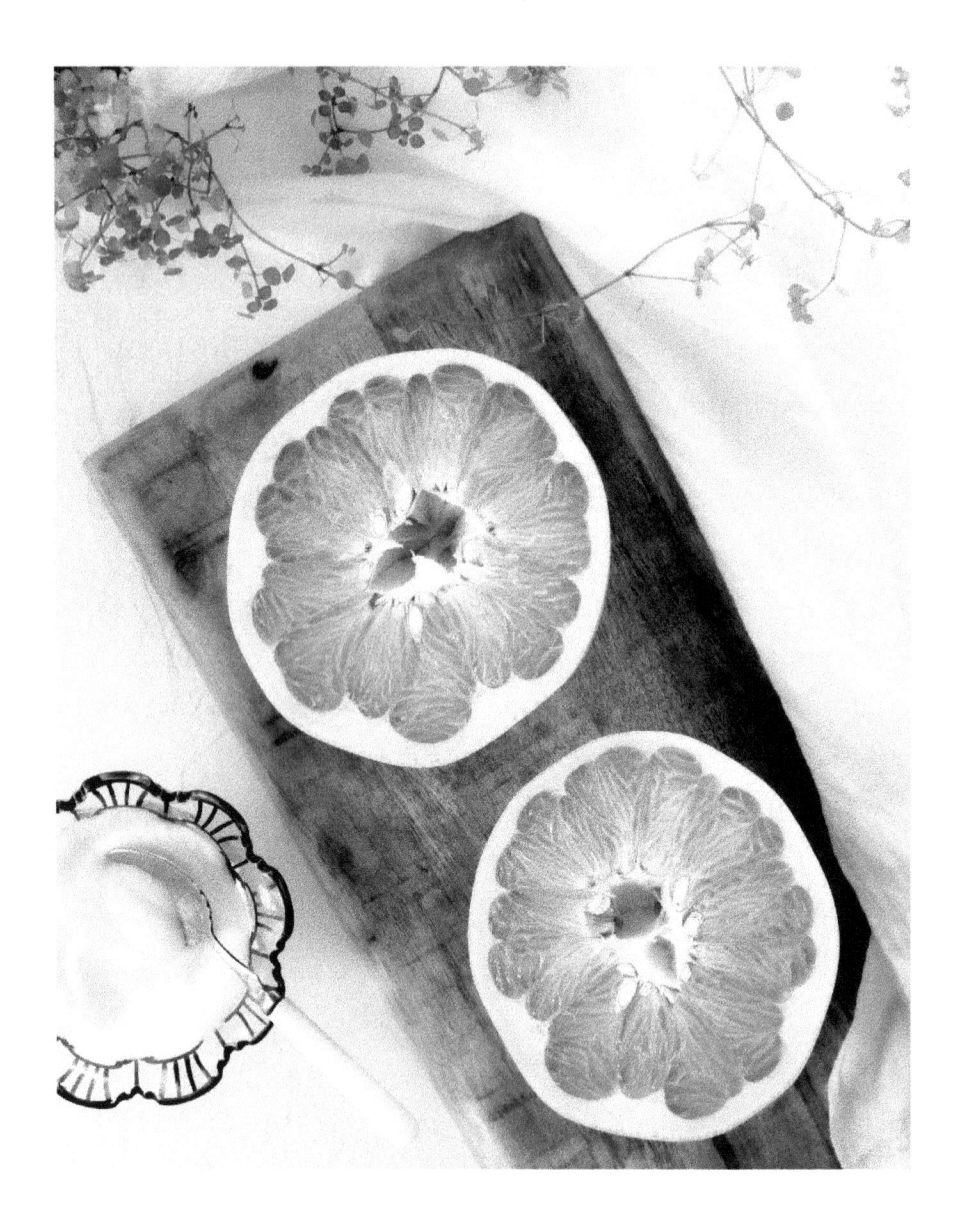

Dinner Recipes

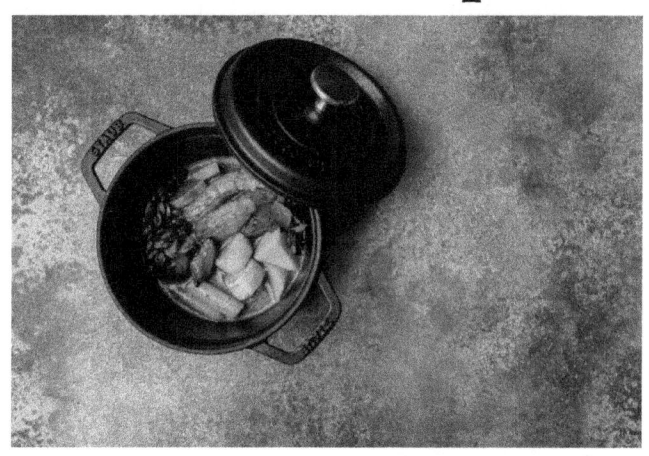

80 Cauliflower Steak Kicking Corn

Preparation: 30 min. Cooking: 60 min. Servings: 6

Ingredients:

2 t. capers, drained 4 scallions, chopped 1 red chili, minced ¼ c. vegetable oil

2 ears of corn, shucked 2 big cauliflower heads Salt and pepper to taste Directions:
Heat the oven to 375 degrees.

Boil a pot of water, about 4 cups, using the maximum heat setting available.

Add corn in the saucepan, cooking approximately 3 minutes or until tender.

Drain and allow the corn to cool, then slice the kernels away from the cob.

Warm 2 tablespoons of vegetable oil in a skillet.

Combine the chili pepper with the oil, cooking for approximately 30seconds.

Next, combine the scallions, sautéing with the chili pepper until soft. Mix in the corn and capers in the skillet and cook for approximately 1 minute to blend the flavors. Then remove from heat. Warm 1 tablespoon of vegetable oil in a skillet. Once warm, begin to place cauliflower steaks to the pan, 2 to 3 at a time. Season to your liking with salt and cook over medium heat for 3 minutes or until lightly browned. Once cooked, slide onto the cookie sheet and repeat step 5 with the remaining cauliflower.

Take the corn mixture and press into the spaces between the florets of the cauliflower.

Bake for 25 minutes. Serve warm and enjoy!
Nutrition: Calories: 153 | Carbohydrates: 15 g | Proteins: 4 g | Fats:10 g

81 Green beans stir fry

Preparation time 30 minutes

Cooking time: 10 minutesServings: 6-8 Ingredients:
1 1/2 pounds of green beans, stringed, chopped into 1 ½-inchpieces

1 large onion, thinly sliced4 star anise (optional)
3 tablespoons avocado oil

1 1/2 tablespoons tamari sauce or soy sauceSalt to taste
3/4 cup water

Direction:

Place a wok over medium heat. Add oil. When oil is heated, addonions and sauté until onions are translucent.

Add beans, water, tamari sauce, and star anise and stir. Cover andcook until the beans are tender.

Uncover, add salt and raise the heat to high. Cook until the waterdries up in the wok. Stir a couple of times while cooking.

82 Mean bean minestrone

Preparation time: 45 minutes Cooking time: 40 minutes Servings: 6
Protein content per serving: 9g Ingredients
1 tablespoon (15 ml) olive oil

1/3 cup (80 g) chopped red onion

4 cloves garlic, grated or pressed

1 leek, white and light green parts, trimmed and chopped (about 4 ounces, or 113 g)

2 carrots, peeled and minced (about 4 ounces, or 113 g) 2 ribs of celery, minced (about 2 ounces, or 57 g)

2 yellow squashes, trimmed and chopped (about 8 ounces, or 227 g) 1 green bell pepper, trimmed and chopped (about 8 ounces, or 227 g)

1 tablespoon (16 g) tomato paste 1 teaspoon dried oregano

1 teaspoon dried basil

⅓ teaspoon smoked paprika

'¼ To ¼ teaspoon cayenne pepper, or to taste

2 cans (each 15 ounces, or 425 g) diced fire-roasted tomatoes 4 cups (940 ml) vegetable broth, more if needed

3 cups (532 g) cannellini beans, or other white beans

2 cups (330 g) cooked farro, or other whole grain or pasta
Salt, to taste
Nut and seed sprinkles, for garnish, optional and to taste

Directions:

In a large pot, add the oil, onion, garlic, leek, carrots, celery, yellow

squash, bell pepper, tomato paste, oregano, basil, paprika, and cayenne pepper. Cook on medium-high heat, stirring often until the vegetables start to get tender, about 6 minutes.

Add the tomatoes and broth. Bring to a boil, lower the heat, cover with a lid, and simmer 15 minutes.

Add the beans and simmer another 10 minutes. Add the farro and simmer 5 more minutes to heat the farro.

Note that this is a thick minestrone. If there are leftovers (which tasteeven better, by the way), the soup will thicken more once chilled.

Add extra broth if you prefer a thinner soup and adjust seasoning if needed. Add nut and seed sprinkles on each portion upon serving, if desired.

Store leftovers in an airtight container in the refrigerator for up to 5 days. The minestrone can also be frozen for up to 3 months.

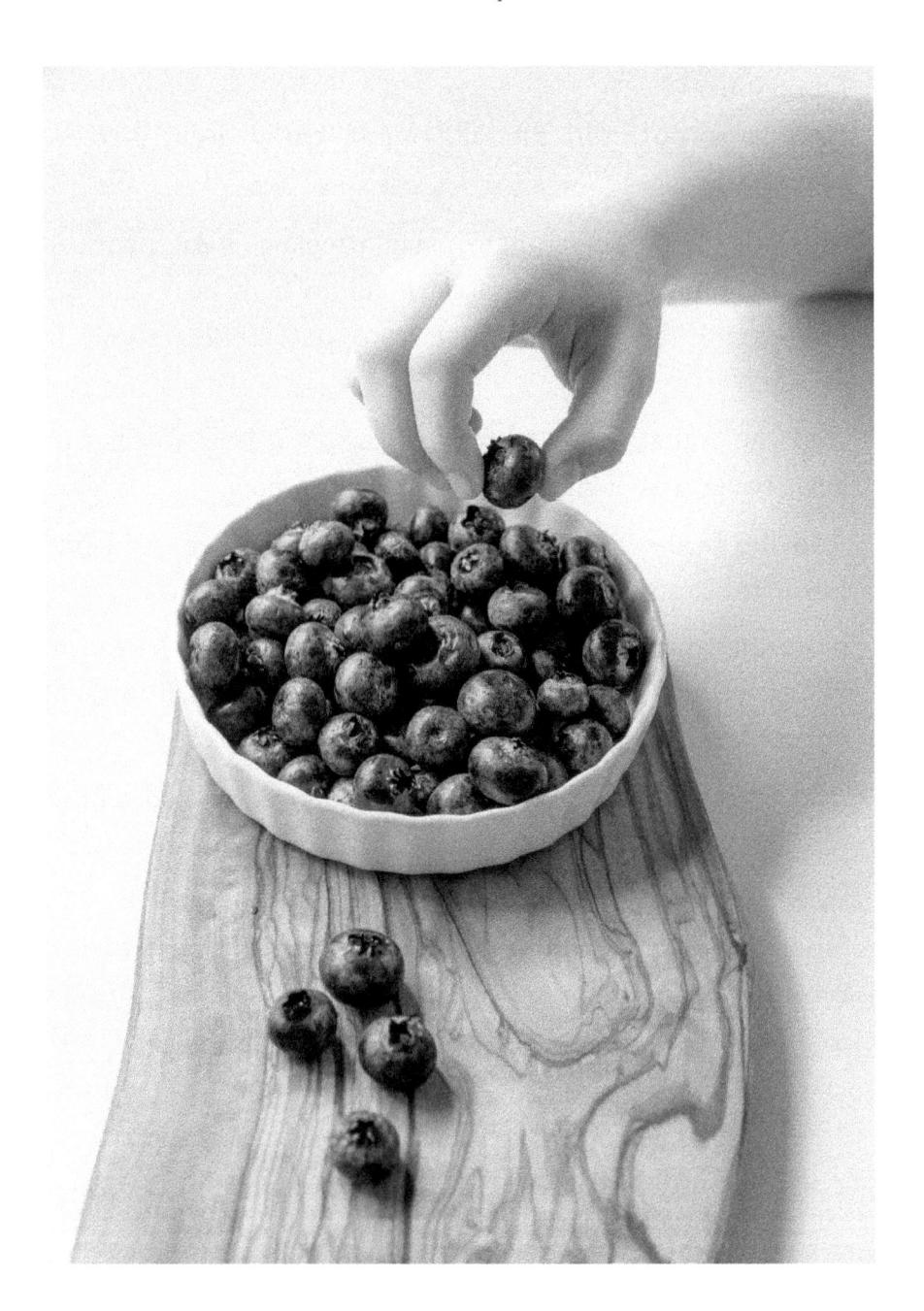

Lunch Recipes

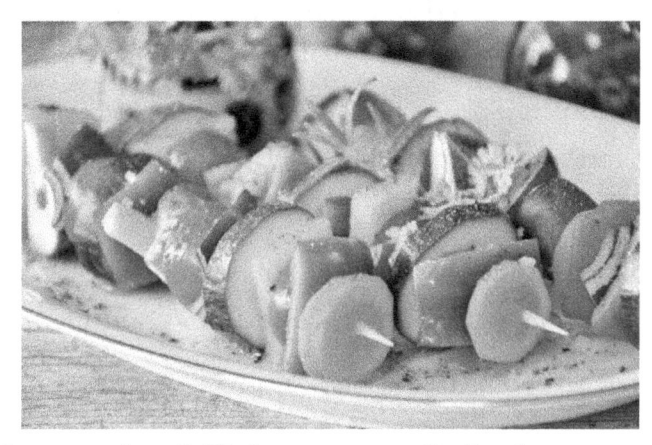

83 Chickpea And Edamame Salad

Preparation Time: 40 minutes Cooking Time: 0 minutes Serving: 4
Ingredients:

For the Salad:

2 tablespoons dried cranberries 1/4 cup (59 grams) diced carrots
3/4 cup (177 grams) edamame soybeans 1/3 cup (78 grams) chopped green pepper 30 ounces (850 grams) cooked chickpeas 1/3 cup (78 grams) chopped red pepper 1/2 teaspoon minced garlic
For the Dressing:

1/4 teaspoon dried oregano 1 teaspoon coconut sugar 1/4 teaspoon dried basil
1/3 teaspoon ground black pepper

1/3 teaspoon salt

1/4 teaspoon dried rosemary 1 teaspoon white vinegar
2 tablespoons grape seed oil 2 tablespoons olive oil

Directions:

Preparethe salad: takealargesaladbowl, place allsalad ingredients in it and then toss until properly mixed.

Preparehe dressing:takeasmall bowl,placealldressing ingredients in it and then whisk until combined.

Drizzle dressing over salad and toss until well mixed.

Place the salad bowl in the refrigerator for at least 30 minutes untilchilled, then serve.

Nutrition: 119.6 Cal; 1.9 g Fat; 0.1 g Saturated Fat; 20.8 g Carbs; 4.8g Fiber; 6 g Protein; 1.1 g Sugar;

84 Cauliflower Salad

Preparation Time: 20 minutes Cooking Time: 15 minutes
Servings: 4
Ingredients:

8 cups cauliflower florets

5 tablespoons olive oil, divided Salt and pepper to taste
1 cup parsley

1 clove garlic, minced

2 tablespoons lemon juice

¼ cup almonds, toasted and sliced 3 cups arugula
2 tablespoons olives, sliced

¼ cup feta, crumbled Direction
Preheat your oven to 425 degrees F.

Toss the cauliflower in a mixture of 1 tablespoon olive oil, salt and pepper. Place in a baking pan and roast for 15 minutes. Put the parsley, remaining oil, garlic, lemon juice, salt and pepper in a blender. Pulse until smooth.

Place the roasted cauliflower in a salad bowl.

Stir in the rest of the ingredients along with the parsley dressing.

Nutrition: Calories: 198 Total fat: 16.5g Saturated fat: 3g Cholesterol: 6mg Sodium: 3mg Potassium: 570mg Carbohydrates: 10.4g Fiber: 4.1g Sugar: 4g Protein: 5.4g

85 Garlic Mashed Potatoes & Turnips

Preparation: 20 minutesCooking: 30 minutes Servings: 8
Ingredients:

1 head garlic 1 teaspoon olive oil lb. turnips, sliced into cubes lb. potatoes, sliced into cubes

½ cup almond milk

½ cup vegan parmesan cheese, grated 1 tablespoon fresh thyme, chopped

1 tablespoon fresh chives, chopped 2 tablespoons vegan butter

Salt and pepper to tasteDirection

Preheat your oven to 375 degrees F. Slice the tip off the garlic head.
Drizzle with a little oil and roast in the oven for 45 minutes.

Boil the turnips and potatoes in a pot of water for 30 minutes or untiltender.

Add all the ingredients to a food processor along with the garlic. Pulse until smooth.

Nutrition: Calories: 141 Total fat: 3.2g Saturated fat: 1.5g Cholesterol: 7mg Sodium: 284mg Potassium: 676mg Carbohydrates: 24.6g Fiber: 3.1g Sugar: 4g Protein: 4.6g

86 Pulled "Pork" Sandwiches

This pulled "pork" is the perfect dish to make ahead. Prepare the mushrooms and coat them in the sauce and then you can store them chilled in the cold-storage box or the icebox. If you prepare a large amount to keep in the icebox, you will always have some on hand for sandwiches, pizza, nachos, or any other vegan-version of popular dishes that might be complemented by pulled "pork".

Preparation time: 40 minutes Cooking Time: 35 minutes
Servings: 3
Ingredients:

King oyster mushrooms* – 4 Barbecue sauce – .25 cup Olive oil – 2 tablespoons Sea salt – .25 teaspoon Garlic, minced – 2 cloves
Cayenne pepper – .25 teaspoon Bread – 6 slices
Directions:

Start by setting your electric cooker to Fahrenheit 400 degrees.

While your electric cooker warms up, clean the mushrooms with a damp paper towel and then use two forks to shred both the caps and stems of the mushrooms into pieces resembling pulled pork. Place

the shredded mushrooms on a kitchen parchment-lined aluminum baking sheet.

Drizzle the mushrooms with half of the olive oil and then toss them with the seasoning and garlic until evenly coated. Allow the oyster mushrooms to roast until slightly crispy and browned about twenty minutes.

In a skillet, add the remaining tablespoon of olive oil, allowing it to warm over midway-elevated. Put the cooked mushrooms in the pan along with the barbecue sauce.

Cook the mushrooms in the sauce while stirring until the sauce is fragrant and warm, about three to five minutes. Top three slices of bread with this concoction and top with the remaining three slices. Cut the sandwiches in half before serving. Note:

*If you can't find king oyster mushrooms, then you can use three heaping cups of regular oyster mushrooms.

Nutrition: Calories 259

87 Coconut zucchini cream

Preparation time: 10 minutes Cooking time: 25 minutes
Servings: 4
Ingredients:

1 pound zucchinis, roughly chopped 2 tablespoons avocado oil

4 scallions, chopped

Salt and black pepper to the taste 6 cups veggie stock
1 teaspoon basil, dried

1 teaspoon cumin, ground 3 garlic cloves, minced
¾ cup coconut cream

1 tablespoon dill, chopped Directions:
Heat up a pot with the oil over medium high heat, add the scallions

and the garlic and sauté for 5 minutes.

Add the rest of the ingredients, stir, bring to a simmer and cook over medium heat for 20 minutes more.

Blend the soup using an immersion blender, ladle into bowls and serve.

Nutrition: calories 160, fat 4, fiber 2, carbs 4, protein 8

88 Zucchini and Cauliflower Soup

Preparation time: 10 minutesCooking time: 25 minutes

Servings: 4Ingredients:

4 scallions, chopped

1 teaspoon ginger, grated2 tablespoons olive oil

1 pound zucchinis, sliced

2 cups cauliflower florets

Salt and black pepper to the taste6 cups veggie stock

1 garlic clove, minced

1 tablespoon lemon juice1 cup coconut cream Directions:

Heat up a pot with the oil over medium heat, add the scallions, ginger and the garlic and sauté for 5 minutes.

Add the rest of the ingredients, bring to a simmer and cook overmedium heat for 20 minutes.

Blend everything using an immersion blender, ladle into soup bowlsand serve.

Nutrition: calories 154, fat 12, fiber 3, carbs 5, protein 4

89 Chard soup

Preparation time: 10 minutes Cooking time: 25 minutes
Servings: 4
Ingredients:

1 pound Swiss chard, chopped

½ cup shallots, chopped 1 tablespoon avocado oil 1 teaspoon cumin, ground

1 teaspoon rosemary, dried 1 teaspoon basil, dried
2 garlic cloves, minced

Salt and black pepper to the taste 6 cups vegetable stock
1 tablespoon tomato passata

1 tablespoon cilantro, chopped Directions:
Heat up a pan with the oil over medium heat, add the shallots and

the garlic and sauté for 5 minutes.

Add the swiss chard and the other ingredients, toss, bring to a simmer and cook over medium heat for 20 minutes more.

Divide the soup into bowls and serve.

Nutrition: calories 232, fat 23, fiber 3, carbs 4, protein 3

90 Eggplant and Olives Stew

Preparation time: 10 minutes Cooking time: 30 minutes
Servings: 4
Ingredients:

1 scallions, chopped

2 tablespoons avocado oil

2 garlic cloves, chopped 1 bunch parsley, chopped
Salt and black pepper to the taste

1 teaspoon basil, dried 1 teaspoon cumin, dried

2 eggplants, roughly cubed

1 cup green olives, pitted and sliced 3 tablespoons balsamic vinegar

½ Cup tomato passata Directions:

Heat up a pot with the oil over medium heat, add the scallions, garlic, basil and cumin and sauté for 5 minutes.

Add the eggplants and the other ingredients, toss, cook over medium heat for 25 minutes more, divide into bowls and serve.

Nutrition: calories 93, fat 1.8, fiber 10.6, carbs 18.6, protein 3.4

Recipes For Main Courses And Single Dishes

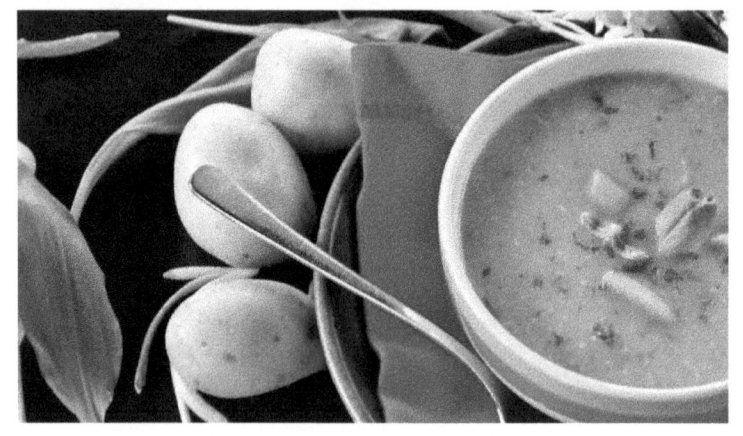

91 Pecan & Blueberry Crumble

Preparation Time: 40 Minutes Cooking Time: 1 Hour
Servings: 6
Calories: 381

Protein: 10 Grams

Fat: 32 Grams

Net Carbs: 20 GramsIngredients:
14 Ounces Blueberries

1 Tablespoon Lemon Juice, Fresh 1 ½ Teaspoon Stevia Powder
3 Tablespoons Chia Seeds

2 Cups Almond Flour, Blanched

¼ Cup Pecans, Chopped 5 Tablespoon coconut Oil 2 Tablespoon Cinnamon Directions:

Mix together your blueberries, stevia, chia seeds and lemon juice, and place it in an iron skillet.

Mix ingredients while spreading it over your blueberries.

Heat your oven to 400, and then transfer it to an oven safe skillet, baking for a half hour.

Interesting Facts: Blueberries: These guys are a delectable treat thatis easily incorporated into many dishes. They are packed with antioxidants and Vitamin C. Bonus: Blueberries have been proven to promote eye health and slow macular degeneration.

92 Rice Pudding

Preparation Time: 1 Hour 35 Minutes Cooking Time: 1 Hour and 30 MinutesServings: 6
Ingredients:

1 Cup Brown Rice

1 Teaspoon Vanilla Extract, Pure

½ Teaspoon Sea Salt, Fine

½ Teaspoon Cinnamon

¼ Teaspoon Nutmeg3 Egg Substitutes
3 Cups Coconut Milk, Light

2 Cups Brown Rice, CookedDirections:
Blend all of your ingredients together before pouring them into a twoquarter dish.

Bake at 300 for ninety minutes before serving.

Interesting Facts: Brown rice is incredibly high in antioxidants and good vitamins. It's relative, 14 white rice is far less beneficial as much of these healthy nutrients get destroyed during the process of milling. You can also opt for red and black rice or wild rice. The meal options for this healthy grain are limitless!

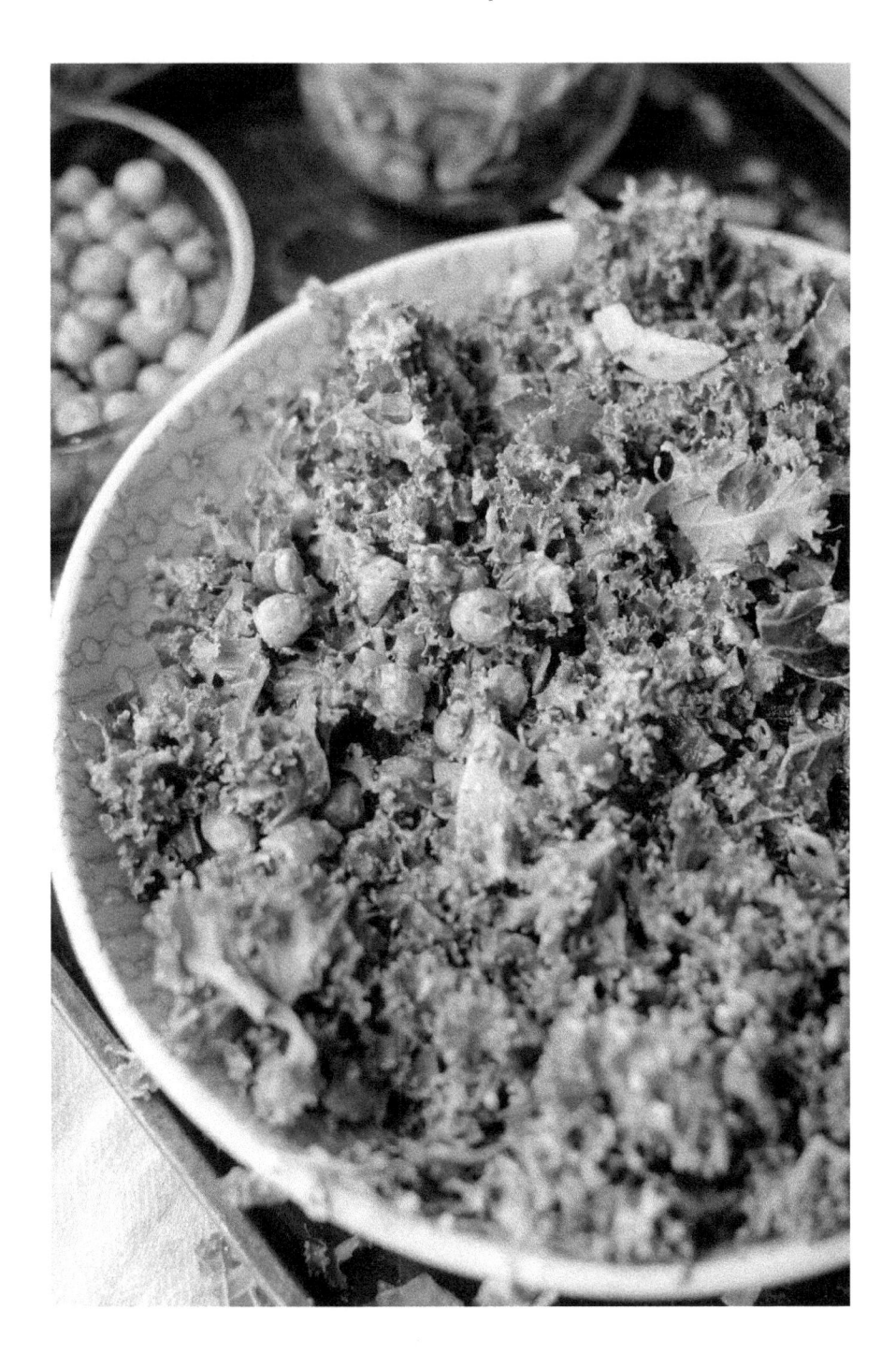

Nutrient-Packed Protein Salads

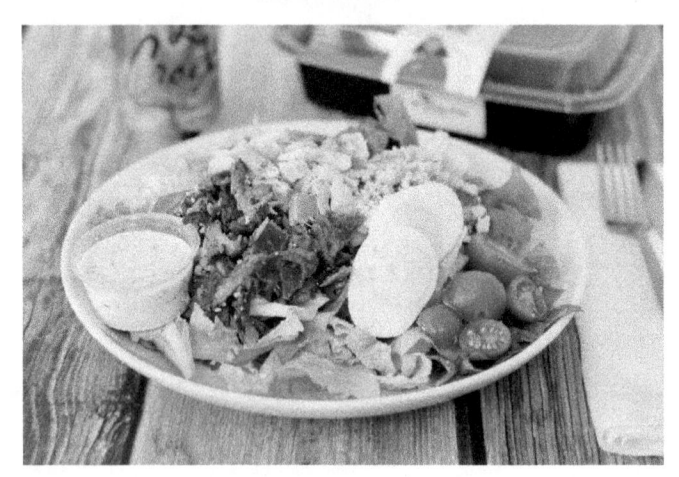

93 Chickpea, Red Kidney Bean And Feta Salad

Preparation time: 5 mins Cooking time: 5 mins Ingredient:

1 can chickpeas

1 can red kidney beans

1 piece small of ginger grated or shredded 1 medium onion diced

2-3 cloves garlic

1 tbsp olive oil

A pinch of red chili flakes

3-4 spring onions green part only, chopped, scallions 1 cup chopped parsley OR coriander I used cilantro Juice of one lemon150 g feta cheese – almost half cup size Salt and Black pepper.

Directions:

Heat 1 tablespoon of olive oil and cook the onion till lightly golden. Do not overdo it and the onions should still be crunchy. Add garlic, ginger and chili and cook till the garlic is fragrant. Set aside to coolso it doesn't melt the feta when you mix it in. Drain the chickpeas and red kidney beans, rinse and place in the salad bowl. Add crumbled feta, spring onion, parsley (or coriander) and lemon juice, season with salt and pepper. Add the cooled onion and garlic mixtureand remaining oil and mix well.

94 Curried Carrot Slaw With Tempeh

Preparation: 10 mins Cooking: 10 mins

Ingredient:

8 ounces tempeh, sliced into triangles 1/4 tsp liquid smoke (optional) 1 1/2 Tbsp maple syrup, grade B

1 tsp extra virgin olive oil or virgin coconut oil 2-3 tsp tamari or 2 tsp soy sauce

1 Tbsp crushed raw walnuts 4 cups shredded carrots

1 small onion, diced 1 Tbsp curry powder

1/4 tsp turmeric powder (for added turmeric power, optional) 1/8 tsp black pepper 2 Tbsp tahini

1/4 cup fresh lemon juice sweet stuff: 1 – 1 1/2 Tbsp maple syrup + an optional handful or raisins

1/2 cup flat leaf parsley, finely chopped + some for garnish

a few pinches of cayenne for heat (optional) salt and pepper for carrot salad – to taste.

Directions:

Warm a skillet up over high heat and add in the coconut or olive oil. When oil is hot, add the tempeh triangles, tamari, maple and liquid smoke. Flip the tempeh around a bit to allow it to absorb the liquid. Cook for about 5 minutes, flipping the tempeh a few times throughout the cooking process. When tempeh is browned and edges blackened a bit, and all liquid absorbed, turn off heat. Sprinkle the walnut pieces and some black pepper over top the tempeh and set pan aside to keep triangles warm in skillet. In a large mixingbowl, add the carrots, tahini, lemon juice, spices, parsley, maple syrup, optional raisins and onion. Toss very well for a few minutes to marinate the carrots with the dressing. For a creamier salad, add another spoonful of tahini. To thin things out and make the salad zestier, add another splash of lemon juice or a teaspoon of apple cider vinegar. Finally, add salt and pepper to the carrot salad totaste. Pour the carrot salad in a large serving bowl and top with the tempeh. Serve right away or place in the fridge to serve in a few hours or up to a day later. The carrots will soften the longer they set in the fridge.

95 Black & White Bean Quinoa Salad

Preparation time: 15 mins Cooking time: 15 mins
Ingredient:

⅓ cup (75 mL) quinoa

1 can (19 oz/540 mL) black beans, drained and rinsed

1 can (19 oz/540 mL) navy beans, drained and rinsed 1 cup (250 mL) diced cucumbers
¼ cup (50 mL) diced red onion

1 jalapeno pepper, seeded and minced (I've never used it and find the dish spicy enough for me, but feel free to add it if you like things hot!)

¼ cup (50 mL) chopped fresh coriander (cilantro)

¼ cup (50 mL) vegetable oil (I use cold pressed extra-virgin olive oil)

2 tbsp (25 mL) lime juice

1 tbsp (15 mL) cider vinegar 1 clove garlic, minced
½ tsp (2 mL) chili powder

1 tsp (5 mL) ground coriander

½ tsp (2 mL) dried oregano

¼ tsp (1 mL) salt

¼ tsp (1 mL) pepper.

Directions:

In saucepan of boiling salted ⅔ C water, cook quinoa until

tender, about 12 minutes. Drain and rinse. Dressing: In large bowl, whisk together oil, lime juice, vinegar, garlic, chili powder, coriander, oregano, salt and pepper. Add quinoa, black beans, navy beans, cucumber, onion, jalapeño pepper and coriander; toss to combine.

96 Greek Salad With Seitan Gyros Strips

Preparation time: 5 mins

Cooking time: 5 mins Ingredient: 4 tomatoes
1 punnet cherry tomatoes

1 1/2 crunchy cucumbers

1 big handful kalamata olives 1/2 Spanish onion finely sliced

1/4 stick of Cheesy mozzarella style cheese. Fresh oregano and mint

1/4 cup good quality extra virgin olive oil

2 Tablespoons vinegar (red wine or balsamic) 1 teaspoon castor sugar

2 teaspoons mixed dried Italian herbs 1 clove finely chopped garlic

2 teaspoon soy sauce salt pepper.

Directions:

In a small frying pan, place gyros strips and fry until slightly blackened on the edges. Leave to cool. Cut up all your veggies roughly and place in a large bowl. Add olives, oregano, mint and chopped cheese. In a jar add all dressing ingredients. Shake well and taste. Combine the cooled gyros strips, salad and dressing and coat well.

97 Chickpea And Edamame Salad

Preparation time: 30 mins

Cooking time: 30 mins

Ingredient: 2 15.5oz each cans chickpea (garbanzo beans) rinsed and drained

3/4 cup edamame soy beans 1/3 cup chopped red pepper 1/3 cup chopped green pepper 1/4 cup diced carrots

3 tablespoons dried cranberries 1 garlic clove minced
Dressing

2 tablespoons grapeseed oil 2 tablespoons olive oil
1 teaspoon white distilled vinegar 1 teaspoon sugar
1/4 teaspoon dried oregano 1/4 teaspoon dried basil
1/4 teaspoon dried rosemary

Salt and pepper Directions:

In a large bowl combine chickpeas, edamame, red pepper, green

pepper, carrots, dried cranberries, minced garlic and set aside. In a small bowl combine grapeseed oil, olive oil, vinegar, sugar, oregano, basil and rosemary. Whisk until blended. Pour dressing over chick peas and gently toss. Season with salt and pepper to taste. Chill for at least 30 minutes for flavors to blend. Serve chilled.

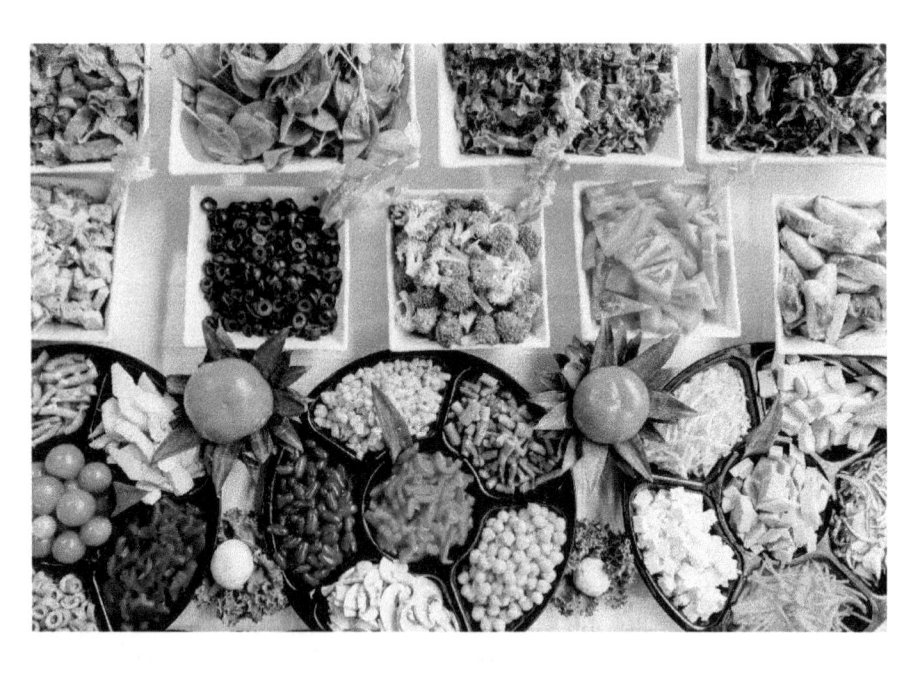

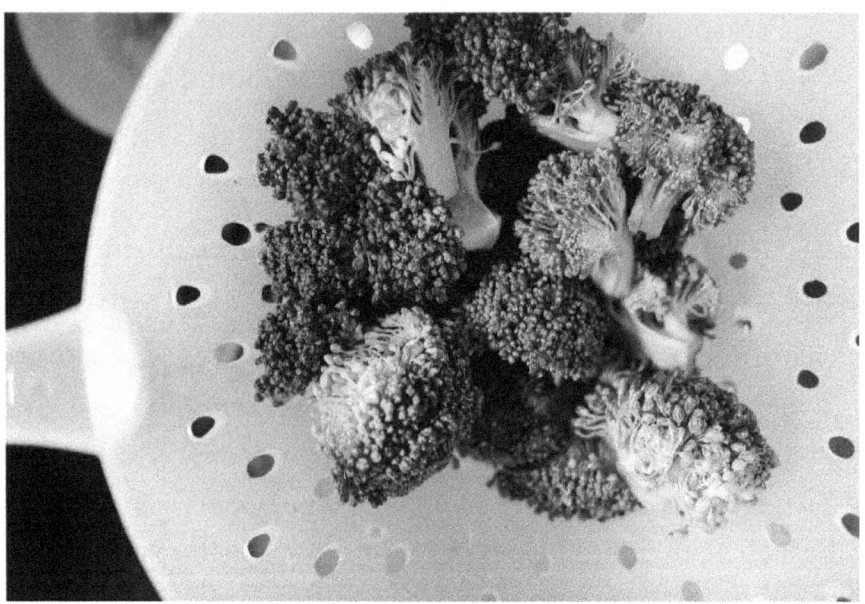

Flavour Boosters (Fish Glazes, Meat Rubs & Fish Rubs)

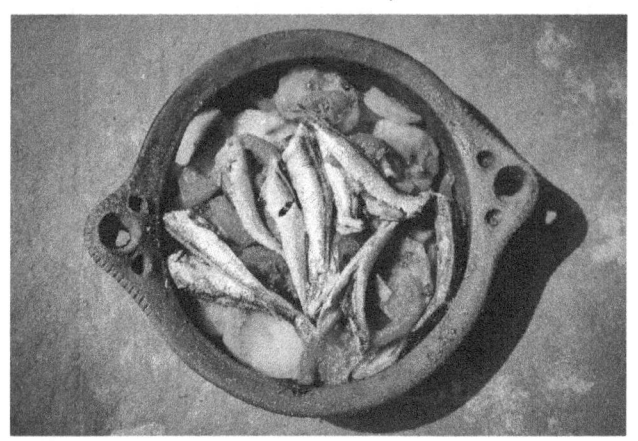

98 Mexican Cocoa Rub

Want to spice up your dry meats with savory Mexican flavors? Try out my classy rub this weekend. Cocoa and espresso powder are a special addition to this Mexican style rub creating soothing spiced aroma.

Preparation Time: 5 min. Cooking Time: 5 min. Servings: 9 tsp.

Ingredients:

Water – 1 tbs.

Cocoa, unsweetened – 1 tsp. Instant espresso powder – 2 tsp. Smoked paprika – 2 tsp.
Olive oil – 1 tsp. Ground cumin – 1 tsp. Salt – ¼ tsp.

Directions:

One by one, mix in all the ingredients in your mixing bowl to makethe cocoa rub. Gently mix all the ingredients using spatula or spoon to form an aromatic rub mixture.

Now, take your choice of meat cut and place it on a firm surface. Brush or rub the freshly made rub on it; pat gently for the rub to stick to the surface. Turn the meat cut and repeat to spice up its other side. Repeat with other meat cuts.

Let your meat cuts adequately season for more rich flavors for a few hours in your refrigerator. Take them out, as they are ready to be cooked or grilled!

99 Juniper Sage Meat Rub

This unique meat rub has been crafted with quality by including numerous healthy herbs such as juniper berries, lay leaf, red pepper, etc. It delivers piney accent to the rub, which ultimately enhances the flavor of your favorite meat cuts.

Preparation Time: 5 min. Cooking Time: 5 min.
Servings: 8 tsp. Ingredients:

Bay leaf – 1 Black peppercorns - 1 tsp. Juniper berries - 2 tsp. Extra-virgin olive oil - 2 tbs. Crushed red pepper - ½ tsp. Kosher salt - ½ tsp.
Minced garlic – 1 clove Minced sage leaves - 6 Directions:

Mix in the bay leaf, red pepper, salt, peppercorns, and berries in your spice blender, grinder or processor to make the juniper rub. Start processing or grinding the mixed spiced on "pulse" mode to ground.

Empty the mixed spice mixture in a bowl; mix in the sage leaves, oil, and garlic. Mix again well.

Now, take your choice of meat cut and place it on a firm surface. Brush or rub the freshly made rub on it; pat gently for the rub to stick to the surface. Turn the meat cut and repeat to spice up its other side. Repeat with other meat cuts.

The freshly rubbed meat is ready to be grilled or cooked!

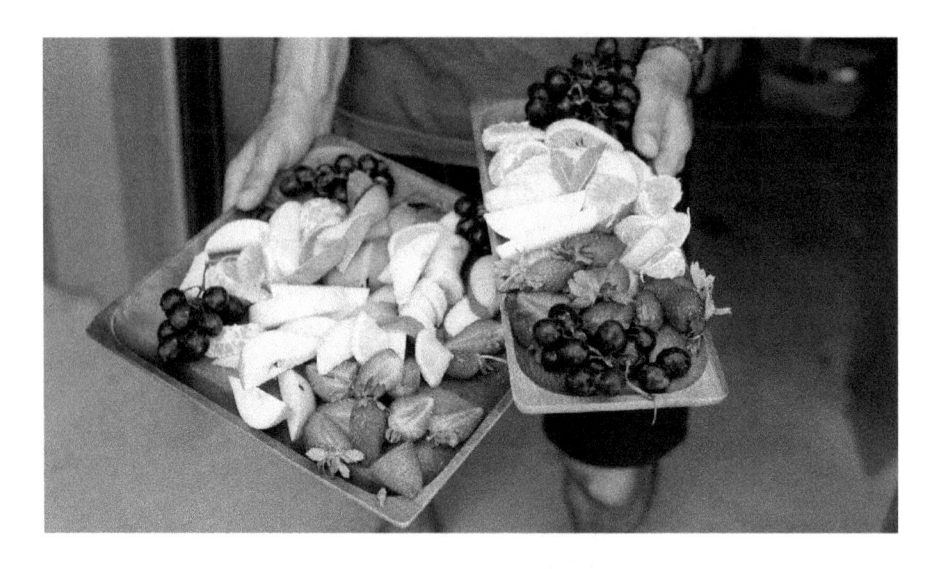

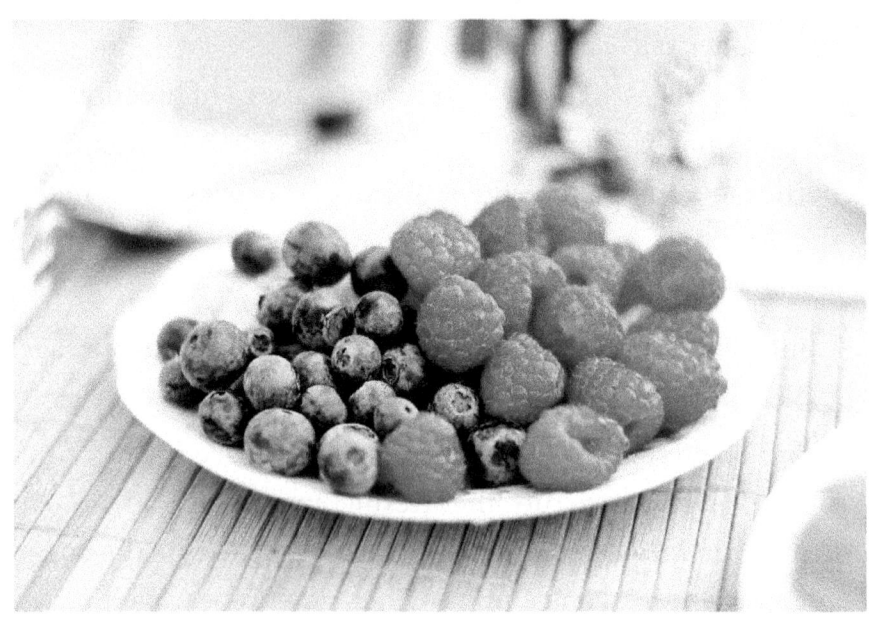

Sauce Recipes

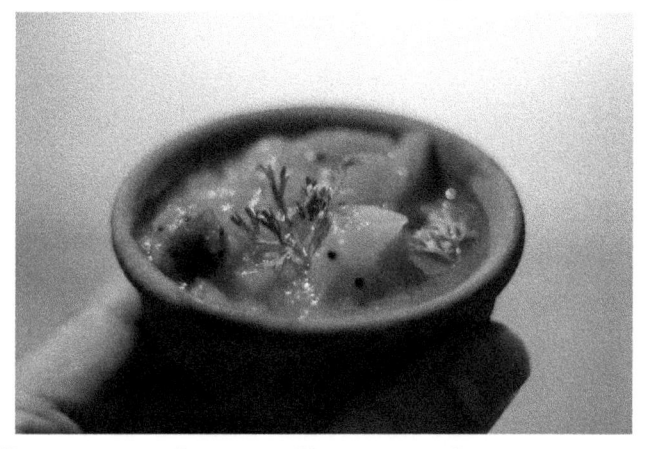

100 Coconut Sugar Peanut Sauce

Preparation time: 5 minutes Cooking time: 5 minute Servings: 1 ½ cups Ingredients

4 tablespoons coconut sugar

6 tablespoons powdered peanut butter 1 tablespoon chili sauce

2 tablespoons liquid aminos

¼ cup of water

1 teaspoon lime juice

½ teaspoon ginger powderDirections:
In a bowl, combine all the ingredients until properly combined. Serve

as a topping for the salad or other dishes.Store in a fridge.